D0848508

# Attacking Animal Diseases

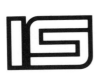

**PAUL R. SCHNURRENBERGER,** D.V.M., M.P.H.
**ROBERT S. SHARMAN,** D.V.M.
**GILBERT H. WISE,** D.V.M.

# Attacking Animal Diseases

## Concepts and Strategies for Control and Eradication

**IOWA STATE UNIVERSITY PRESS,** AMES, IOWA

**Paul R. Schnurrenberger** was a graduate of the Ohio State University School of Veterinary Medicine and received a masters degree in public health from the University of Pittsburgh. He was professor and department head at Ahmadu Bello University, Zaria, Nigeria; a Fulbright scholar at Murdoch University, Perth, Australia; and at the time of his death in 1984 was professor of public health at the Auburn University School of Veterinary Medicine. He was a diplomate of the American College of Veterinary Preventive Medicine.

**Robert S. Sharman** is a graduate of the Alabama Polytechnic Institute (Auburn University) School of Veterinary Medicine. He has served in eradication programs in Mexico with the U.S. Department of Agriculture. Since retiring as Deputy Administrator, Veterinary Services, USDA, he has served as U.S. Commissioner for an eradication program in Mexico and on the faculty of the Auburn University School of Veterinary Medicine. He is a diplomate of the American College of Veterinary Preventive Medicine.

**Gilbert H. Wise** is a graduate of the Michigan State University School of Veterinary Medicine. He was in the Veterinary Corps, U.S. Army and a private practitioner before joining the U.S. Department of Agriculture, where he served in a variety of animal health and consumer protection assignments. At the time of his retirement he was Associate Administrator, Animal and Plant Health Inspection Service, USDA. He is a diplomate of the American College of Veterinary Preventive Medicine.

© 1987 Iowa State University Press, Ames, Iowa 50010
All rights reserved

Composed by Iowa State University Press
Printed in the United States of America

No part of this book may be reproduced in any form or by any electronic or mechanical means, including information storage and retrieval systems, without written permission from the publisher, except for brief passages quoted in a review.

First edition, 1987

**Library of Congress Cataloging-in-Publication Data**

Schnurrenberger, Paul R., 1929–
    Attacking animal diseases.

    Bibliography: p.
    Includes index.
    1. Veterinary public health.    I. Sharman, Robert S.    II. Wise, Gilbert H., 1921–
III. Title.
SF740.S37    1987    636.089´44    87–2825
ISBN 0-8138-0156-7

OLSON LIBRARY
NORTHERN MICHIGAN UNIVERSITY
MARQUETTE, MICHIGAN 49855

**Dedicated to the memory of**
**PAUL R. SCHNURRENBERGER, D.V.M., M.P.H.** (1929–1984)

# CONTENTS

# PREFACE

PREPARATION for this publication began nearly 40 years ago when the authors were first exposed to the rigors of animal disease eradication programs in the field. Without formal training in program operation, they were thrust into operational situations with only limited literature references to supplement the anecdotal information garnered on occasion from more experienced workers.

There has been little improvement since that time. Schools of veterinary medicine virtually ignore the topic in their undergraduate curricula, graduate programs focus more on sophisticated technology than on program planning and operational problems, and agency training concentrates on program minutiae and managerial philosophy. The forest remains hidden through focussing on the trees.

Acutely aware of this void through having survived it, the authors have compiled this volume, both for neophytes entering the field of disease control and for veterans of eradication campaigns. While it is the authors' conviction that the principles of large-scale animal disease control and eradication apply throughout the world, the tactical application of these principles must vary widely due to economic, cultural, and environmental differences.

This publication is oriented toward the Western Hemisphere, with considerable reliance on experiences in the United States and Canada. To date, these two countries have had the widest coverage in the hemisphere in both numbers and scope of animal health programs, particularly those of disease eradication.

Numerous people have provided information for this publication. Much of the material was presented first as a seminar at Auburn University, Alabama, in 1979, with participants and speakers coming from various areas of the Western Hemisphere. The seminar was presented again with a reduced faculty in Georgetown, Guyana, in August 1980 and was sponsored by the Inter-American Institute for Cooperation on Agriculture and the Pan American Health Organization. The participants came from the Caribbean community.

Written drafts of the papers presented at these seminars were used as a basic source of information for this volume. Few of those who made the original contributions had an opportunity to consult with one another in advance, resulting in some duplication of information. Portions of the basic papers, while serving well for oral presentation, needed extensive revision for publication. There was also a need to transpose certain subject matter to reinforce the essence of several chapters. For reasons of continuity and breadth of coverage, material has been added by the authors. Therefore it is not possible to credit each chapter with a specific author. However, we do wish to recognize and thank the following individuals who presented material at the original seminars for contributing original thoughts, experience, and long hours of preparation of much of the written and oral material that is the foundation for this book. (The titles are those at the time contributions were made; for those who were retired at that time, the position given is their last official title before retirement.)

**Pedro N. Acha,** Acting Director
Pan American Zoonoses Center
Buenos Aires, Argentina

**J. Lee Alley,** State Veterinarian
Dept. of Agriculture and Industries
Montgomery, Ala.

**Franz C. Alexander,** Animal Health
Specialist
Inter-American Institute for Cooperation
on Agriculture
Georgetown, Guyana

**R. J. Anderson,** Associate Administrator
(retired)
Agricultural Research Service, USDA
Marshall, Tex.

**Abraham Arce**
Potomac, Md.

**J. J. Callis,** Director
Plum Island Animal Disease Center
Greenport, N.Y.

**C. C. Christenberry,** Regional
Epidemiologist
U.S. Dept. of Agriculture
Auburn, Ala.

**Fred Clayton**
Residue Evaluation Program,
U.S. Dept. of Agriculture
Washington, D.C.

**Paul Doby,** Superintendant
Division of Meat, Poultry, and Livestock
Inspection
Illinois Dept. of Agriculture
Springfield, Ill.

**Robert Hanson,** Professor and Chairman
Dept. of Veterinary Science
University of Wisconsin
Madison, Wis.

**Richard O. Hayes,** Technical Program
Director
Frank E. Basil, Inc.
Fort Collins, Colo.

**William T. Hubbert,** Professional
Development Staff
U.S. Dept. of Agriculture
Beltsville, Md.

**Frank J. Mulhern,** Director
Animal Health, Inter-American Institute
for Cooperation on Agriculture
Crofton, Md.

Victor Nettles, Leader
Diagnostic Section, Southeastern
    Cooperative Wildlife Disease Study
Athens, Ga.

Richard E. Omohundro, Director
    (retired)
Emergency Programs, Veterinary
    Services, APHIS, USDA
Littleton, Colo.

Richard L. Parker, Chief
Bureau of Epidemiology, South Carolina
    Dept. of Health and Environmental
    Control
Columbia, S.C.

Gustavo Reta Petterson, Sub-Secretary of
    Agriculture
Secretariat of Agriculture and Hydraulic
    Resources
Mexico City, Mexico

John Richardson, Director
Office of Biosafety, Centers for Disease
    Control
Atlanta, Ga.

Ronald Schultz, Professor
Dept. of Pathobiological Sciences
University of Wisconsin
Madison, Wis.

John Shook, Chief Animal Health and
    State Veterinarian, Animal Health
    and Consumer Services
Annapolis, Md.

B. C. Swindle, Senior Staff Veterinarian
    (retired)
Import/Export Staff, Veterinary Services,
    APHIS, USDA
Lakeland, Fla.

Gilbert Trevino, Professor
Dept. of Veterinary Pathology
Texas A & M University
College Station, Tex.

# Attacking Animal Diseases

# 1

## Introduction

MODERN SOCIETIES CONSIST of a variety of specialized groups, each most familiar with its own work and interests and not too informed about those of other groups. Any large-scale effort involving a wide range of total society, including disease control programs, must be structured in a way that recognizes the many levels and types of understanding involved in a project. Health programs depend not only on scientific and technical knowledge, but also on skill in identifying the variety of political, economic, and cultural interests that will be caught up in the campaign and in melding these varied viewpoints into unified support.

While no program will succeed without adequate scientific knowledge and effective application of technical procedures, any program adopted and pursued solely on a technical basis will fail. Health professionals cannot operate in isolation. Successful disease control or eradication is both a science and an art, and the artistry lies in an ability to orchestrate the application of knowledge in a manner acceptable to many specialized interest groups.

The purpose of this publication is to present a broad view of the conceptual, historical, and operational factors bearing on large-scale public programs to control or eradicate significant animal disease. Definition of these terms is provided as a foundation for reviewing the material in this volume.

*Significant disease* — a disease causing, or capable of causing, major economic or public health damage at a level affecting the general public.

Historically, determination of the amount of damage from a disease has been made from a combination of haphazard observations of losses and speculation on how such losses might be magnified should the agent continue to spread. While more definitive measurement systems have now become available, few diseases are routinely monitored on a comprehensive basis due to the high costs and the consequent low priority such activities receive.

As a result, close attention to obtaining specific data on occurrence and loss from disease usually comes only after the disease has become "significant" in the mind of the public by means other than orderly measurement. For these reasons, animal diseases that cause dramatic economic loss, such as foot-and-mouth disease or hog cholera, are seen as significant. Losses from chronic parasitism or low-grade enteric infections may be large, but the diseases are not perceived to be as significant as those that kill quickly or result in large numbers of acutely ill animals.

Diseases that can affect human as well as nonhuman animals are perceived as significant in similar fashion; those such as rabies and plague, which kill a large percentage of infected people, have historically inspired fear and even panic. Less dramatic zoonoses, such as salmonellosis, have not caused significant public concern and, consequently, have not been the target of major control efforts in most countries.

It is important to recognize that authority to determine the significance of a disease has not rested solely, or even primarily, with health officials. With improved aids for mass diagnostic screening and the growing use of orderly economic models, health authorities can now acquire more definitive information to determine disease significance. The point remains, however, that significance is a subjective term that varies over time and space.

*Disease control program* – an organized effort on a regional, national, or greater basis to reduce incidence of, or losses from, a significant disease to a level that does not have a major impact on the general public.

Control means to exercise a restraining, regulatory, or governing influence. There is a marked difference in purpose, concept, and technique between disease control and agent eradication; however, the two are often regarded by laymen as differing in degree rather than kind. Control is directed toward easing the impact of a disease. Eradication is focused on elimination of an agent. While a planned program to eradicate an established agent will often have an initial period devoted to reducing incidence through control measures prior to moving into eradication procedures, this is to be differentiated from a program strictly limited to disease control.

Conceptually, the primary difference between these two approaches is one of endpoint. Eradication presumes elimination of the disease agent from the political jurisdiction sponsoring the program. In a purely control effort it is understood from the outset that the agent will not be eliminated, that some level of infection will remain, and that control costs will continue indefinitely after the desired level of control has been reached.

Procedurally, this means that options may be broader in a purely control program than in the early phases of an eradication effort. Examples include procedures for handling infected herds or individuals and whether vaccines can be used.

A control program usually does not require the urgency that is characteristic of an eradication campaign. Therefore, in control situations, it is possible to provide an extended time period for neutralizing infected individuals, with greater flexibility in techniques and timing in dealing with infected groups. Since indemnities are absent or restricted in most control programs, this flexibility is used to maintain owner cooperation. As a control program presumes some level of continuing infection, vaccines that may cause postvaccination diagnostic or clinical complications may have a place in a control program, although such vaccines would be unacceptable in final eradication efforts.

It should not be construed that control is necessarily a second-best approach to attacking a problem. In some instances, a sound control program may be the only politically or technically feasible alternative. For example, rabies control in domestic animals is a worthwhile control program in countries where the existence of rabies virus in wild species precludes eradication.

*Disease eradication program* — an organized effort to eliminate a significant disease agent from the area involved so that no further outbreaks occur unless reintroduced from the outside and so that specific immunization or treatment procedures are no longer needed.

Eradication means to pull out by the roots, to extirpate. In terms of disease eradication programs, differences of understanding do not arise from the general concept but over questions of how and when to decide the agent has been eradicated. Those who do not perceive the conceptual difference between disease control and eradication often assume that eradication is no more than a fortunate outcome of control. This view is not conducive to maximum public benefit from health programs. Health professionals must be a resource for clearly expressing differences in concept and technique between control and eradication. Gelfand (1973) listed eradication, death, and pregnancy as the three words in medicine that always denote totality. He further ascribed a qualitative difference to control and eradication: control is concerned with up to the first 99.9% of the cases, whereas eradication is interested only in the last 0.1%.

From a procedural standpoint, the difference between a proper concept of eradication and one that presumes that eradication is merely the fortuitous result of a control program is largely concerned with the level of work needed to achieve true eradication. In a true eradication program, as confirmed outbreaks become less frequent and disappear there is increased investment in the search for residual infection. Against a long-established disease, intensive (and expensive) active surveillance for a year or more after the last confirmed case is necessary before a declaration of final eradication is supportable. The duration of this period varies with the area size, sophistication and sensitivity of the surveillance system, and the epidemiology of the target disease.

This type of search is not characteristic of the concluding phases of a control program, for these programs are not aimed at searching out every vestige of infection. This difference, in terms of final search cost, was illustrated during the hog cholera eradication program in the United States. In the middle years of the program, while the country was moving from the early, or control, phases into the final eradication phases, over 3000 confirmed cases were found, at an average program cost of $13,578 per case. In the final 7 years (1971–1977), when cases were few and the search for infection was the most intensive in the program, only 364 confirmed outbreaks were found, at a program cost of $217,000 per case (USDA 1981).

The comparative economic benefits of eradication and control also differ significantly. As disease control means that some level of infection remains, indefinite, continuing expense is required to prevent a resurgence. Depending on the disease, these costs can include continued immunization, diagnostic screening to monitor disease levels, or regular need for pesticide application. If eradication is erroneously defined only as absence of epidemic disease without including the continuing expense of perpetual protective measures, much of the real economic benefit of eradication is lost. It is important for program planners to identify realistically the goal of any proposed program, so that both procedures and benefits can be analyzed accordingly.

In addition to the preceding definitions, there is a need to define two epidemiologic terms, *incidence* and *prevalence,* that help to describe the risk of exposure to a communicable agent.

*Incidence* — the number of new cases having their onset during a given time. Incidence equals increase (or decrease).

*Prevalence* — a measure of the total number of cases present at a given point in time. Prevalence equals present.

# 2

# Humans and Disease, Distance, and Time

ALTHOUGH HUMANS have been treating diseases since prehistoric times, successful disease control and eradication programs are relatively recent developments in history. These programs have been directed against living agents capable of producing unusual damage, and except for the relatively recent addition of some significant noninfectious diseases (chemical poisoning, industrial pollution), there is no reason to expect this will change. The list of epidemic diseases deserving attention remains far greater than scheduled efforts at control or eradication.

In confronting an infectious disease or parasitic condition in a large host population, we face a living opponent — an adversary that, for survival, must somehow adjust to its host environment, including any changes in that environment resulting from attempts at control or eradication. Recent examples of this adjustment to change caused by human intervention include resistance to penicillin developed by strains of *Neisseria gonorrheae* and *Staphylococcus aureus*.

No life form can be successful unless it can exist within its environment. The struggle for survival by adjusting to a changing environment is as characteristic of living pathogens as for any other form of life. This process, presumably, is as old as life itself. Since infectious diseases result from living agents, it is evident that no disease agent would persist long if it killed 100% of its hosts so quickly that the agent also could not survive. Even though rabies is described as 100% fatal in all species, aggressiveness with frequent biting and tropism of rabies virus for salivary glands provide ample opportunity for the spread of the infecting organism. These two characteristics are far more important than an occasional survivor (Fekadu et al. 1981).

The recent history of African swine fever (ASF) also illustrates this capability for change. Early in the twentieth century, Montgomery (1921), working in Kenya, described a devastating disease in domestic swine. In the outbreaks he studied, herd mortality was 98.9% — hardly encouraging for the future of

7

swine production or, apparently, for the survival of the virus. He also observed that the disease occurred on farms where domestic swine had contact with wild warthogs and bush pigs, species later found to be healthy carriers of ASF virus. With this knowledge, East African pig raisers adopted a policy that was a combination of fencing out wild species and destroying infected domestic herds to prevent ASF virus from cycling in domestic swine.

However, with movement of the disease across Africa and into Portugal and Spain, the ASF virus adjusted to a new environment in generations of domestic swine. Mortality decreased and the problem of chronic or clinically inapparent infections arose. The virus adapted to its new host, markedly enhancing its ability to survive.

The concept of a living, changing opponent is vital to success in large-scale disease eradication operations. Speed of action is essential if a disease agent is to eradicated, especially if found in a previously unexposed host population.

Human efforts to control disease in domestic animals, a very recent intrusion into this natural struggle, are a part of the development of agriculture, a process that has been called the most significant event in the history of humankind (Leakey and Lewin 1977).

For 2 million years our immediate ancestors were hunters and gatherers, moving continually from place to place. Their survival depended upon their skills and understanding the natural world about them but did not include significant interference in the evolution of that world.

Modern humans, *Homo sapiens sapiens,* the only surviving human species for the last 30,000 years, were also hunter-gatherers until about 12,000 years ago. They succeeded in finding their way over most of the world during those wandering days. Populations were small, as our predecessors could not increase in numbers beyond the carrying capacity of the natural world.

Then humans learned, in many parts of the world, to control production of food through agriculture. For the first time humans were significantly altering the natural world for their benefit and had a surplus of food beyond their immediate needs. By 5000 B.C. several wild animal species had been domesticated; sheep, goats, cattle, and pigs were a part of agriculture in the Near East. Humans learned by observation and selection how to alter formerly wild plants and animals to produce varieties better suited to domestication and their personal needs.

This revolution has been very rapid. In only 12,000 years humans have changed from a hunting-gathering life-style that had existed for millions of years to one absolutely dependent on controlled agriculture. The human population has exploded from an estimated 10 million to over 4000 million. The surviving hunter-gatherers exist today only on the fringes of human society, usually in areas where the natural environment is too forbidding to permit the practice of agriculture. Humanity could not survive in today's large numbers without controlled food production.

For most of this agricultural era, humans did not understand the consequences of environmental manipulation. The concentration of domesticated animals and plants allowed, or even encouraged, a similar concentration of pathogens affecting these species. Cultivation of plants and animals increased the carrying capacity of the environment not only for humans, but also for the parasites of all domesticated species. People engaged in agriculture, which still includes most of the world's population, have been contending with this reality ever since.

It is only in the last few generations that we have begun to understand the mechanisms through which diseases operate and been able, in any informed way, to move beyond superstition and empirical remedies in handling the impact of disease. An appreciation of the vast time over which life forms evolved and of their patterns for survival assists in the understanding of why disease functions as it does in the altered environment created by agriculture.

Historically, disease agents have migrated with humanity and their animals. During the centuries when travel was slow and difficult, and trading in animals and animal products was limited, infectious agents moved slowly. For example, rinderpest virus apparently traveled west from China with Mongol invaders, reaching western Asia about 2000 years ago. The virus then took over four centuries to move the relatively short distance into Europe, when it accompanied the invasion of Attila. Once in Europe, rinderpest plagued war-torn areas for over 1000 years until it was eliminated in the late 1800s. Now, with rapid transit by land, sea, and air, as well as worldwide trade in a variety of animal products, the protection against the spread of infectious organisms afforded by spoilage, time, and distance has been reduced. Within the twentieth century alone, ASF has spread from East Africa to South and West Africa, Europe, the Caribbean, and South America.

Even before the work of Pasteur and Koch and the subsequent explosion of knowledge concerning disease, observation of the association of the introduction of disease with animal importation resulted in the beginnings of quarantine and control systems. Slow sea voyages provided a long, natural "quarantine" period for live animals, and a disease in the incubative stage at the start of the voyage was likely to be fatal or evident upon inspection at destination. Land movement of livestock was on foot and proceeded slowly over the few trails or roads available. As opposed to the isolation aboard ship, however, land movement resulted in the possibility of spreading disease agents along the route of travel; obviously, additional controls were needed. In 1795, for example, the North Carolina Legislature forbade driving cattle into the state from the south for fear of introducing disease — possibly bovine babesiosis (cattle-tick fever).

The explosion of scientific and technical knowledge that commenced in the latter half of the nineteenth century changed the patterns of trade and increased opportunities for the spread of pathogens: steam replaced sails for sea travel; regions, formerly weeks or months apart, were separated by only hours or days with the coming of railroads; the industrial revolution created many new commercial processes and products that could be distributed quickly and widely, including products of animal origin. These changes, coupled with expanded studies of the mechanisms of disease occurrence, resulted in altered awareness, as illustrated by recently changed perceptions of foot-and-mouth disease (FMD).

Prior to the late 1800s due to the relatively low mortality and rarity of lengthy serious illness, the full impact of the long-term economic loss from FMD was not appreciated. Understanding these costs grew as research elicited and clarified the pattern of the disease, established where the virus could be found in infected animals, and identified conditions under which the virus could survive in products from such animals.

Apparent changes in the method of dispersal began to be noted. For example, all four introductions of FMD virus into the United States between 1870 and 1902 were attributed to cattle imported from infected countries. From 1902 through 1929, however, all five introductions of the disease apparently were due to contaminated materials, vaccines, or ships' garbage brought ashore and fed to swine.

Altered commercial trade practices added new risks. FMD virus is inactivated rapidly in carcass muscle by lactic acid formation; however, rapidly freezing infected meat prevents this pH reduction and infectivity is retained. This necessitated a new look at the risk of disease from trading frozen meat as opposed to shipping chilled carcasses that are allowed to age unfrozen. The picture was complicated further when it was discovered that less lactic acid formation occurs in pork than in beef.

Information of this type also began to accumulate for other diseases and demonstrated a need for controls over imported animal products in addition to the quarantine measures already in effect for imported animals.

This brought a new dimension to disease prevention. Controls over animal products are, in many ways, more difficult to define and administer than those over international traffic in the animals themselves. Such items are diverse and result from a variety of industrial processes, some of which may reduce disease risk to a negligible level, whereas others do not significantly change the danger. Commercial interests have little understanding of disease or the impact of pathogen introduction and often resist what they perceive as bureaucratic obstacles to trade. The research needed to establish a scientific basis for proper controls is expensive.

The risk of spreading disease increases when distance becomes of little consequence and time in transit can be measured in hours. Within a few hours jet aircraft from any part of the world can reach the interior of any country. Huge, well-constructed shipboard containers discourage complete inspection of animal products at the port of entry. Traditional concepts of quarantine and control systems are now insufficient; oceans, mountains, deserts, swamps, and rivers no longer provide effective barriers. Although most animal disease control and eradication programs continue to be carried out on a country-by-country basis, the overall concept of animal disease now needed is multinational rather than national. Political boundaries are not barriers to disease, and political and economic considerations that may favor increased trade with selected countries may have little to do with the realities of disease risk.

As a result, continuing exchange of information between health authorities is now needed for the safe flow of commerce. Importing countries have a responsibility to require as much information as is appropriate from an animal health standpoint before approving the entry of any potentially dangerous animal or animal product. It is not enough for an importing country to know that a virus vaccine produced in another country is efficacious; it also is important for the importing country to not only know the origin and subsequent history of the seed virus used in vaccine production, but also to know whether or not extraneous disease agents are present. To protect long-term export trade, producing countries need to recognize that providing full factual data on the health aspects of exports is as much a part of the transaction as providing the type and quality of animal or animal product agreed upon.

Mutual confidence depends on a continuing exchange of information between health authorities in all countries. Ongoing publication of statistical data on diseases and populations, supplemented by prompt notification of unusual or emergency situations, is necessary for any exporting country that hopes to retain the confidence of its trading partners.

Collection, organization, and dissemination of health information are carried out by several international organizations. The World Health Organization (WHO), the Food and Agriculture Organization (FAO), and the International Office of Epizootics (OIE) publish periodic statistical compilations of reports supplied by participating countries worldwide (The Animal Disease Yearbook), as well as narrative accounts of specific situations. In the Western Hemisphere, the Pan American Health Organization (PAHO) has long been a source of information about animal health, as has more recently, the Inter-American Institute for Cooperation on Agriculture (IICA).

Information disseminated by any of these organizations can only be as good as the accuracy of the data submitted by member countries. Much of this data is limited, and it seldom reflects the entire picture due to difficulty in obtaining funds to support disease surveillance. However, the international reports, when read in the context of their limitations, provide a foundation for comparisons over time and one on which to build a world view of disease occurrence.

While the need for a world view may seem remote to professionals confronting local problems during their early careers, the value is apparent to anyone reaching the national staff level in a health organization. Therefore, career development should include training that imbues a concept of disease that moves beyond local or national boundaries.

On a nation-by-nation basis, eradication of a variety of animal diseases has been achieved. In some instances a combination of national efforts has led to regional eradication: contagious bovine pleuropneumonia and rinderpest from Europe, and FMD has been stamped out in North America each time it has gained entry. Recently, in response to the increased speed of disease spread, the self-interest of unaffected but threatened countries has led to more organized regional attacks. The elimination of ASF from the Dominican Republic and Haiti involved coordinated support from outside the affected nations.

Still, FMD persists to some degree in Europe and throughout most of South America. The regional eradication campaign involving all countries in a common effort, has to date not been possible, although it seems probable that this is the optimum solution to a continuing and costly endemic problem.

The isolated island protected from outside invaders by virtue of inaccessability is no longer a guarantee of freedom from military attack or the entry of disease. Since the authority to act is, and presumably will continue to be, vested in national rather than international bodies, cooperative multinational actions rather than truly international programs appear to be the most realistic concept in approaching the regional needs of animal disease control or eradication. In this situation, each country in the group must have a compelling self-interest for acting in concert with the efforts of others. If a common interest is not present, it would be an illusion to expect full participation.

In the Western Hemisphere, the nations from Canada south through Panama have maintained a loosely defined but universally accepted policy that reflects a regional "island" concept regarding exotic pests and diseases. This is reflected in several organizations and programs: the Interregional Organization for Livestock and Agricultural Health, the Inter-American Cattlemens Confederation, the cooperative animal health programs, the cooperative plant health programs, and the interchange of incidence information and diagnostic capability.

Agricultural self-interest has resulted in acceptance of the need to protect this island bounded by the Arctic to the north, oceans on either side, and the narrowing land mass touching South America. But there are needs other than protection from agricultural diseases and pests. Recently, pressure has been felt on the southern border of this territory that has led to differences between animal health interests and others primarily concerned with opening a land route from one end of the hemisphere to the other.

Plans to complete the one remaining section of the Pan-American highway through the Darien Gap, a hot, humid, and sparsely populated forest area astride the Panamanian-Columbian border, have raised this issue. There are virtually no trails, roads, or clearings in the area that currently (1984) measures about 50 by 50 miles.

Because of its geographic and climatic situation, this small area has been looked upon by those to the north as a natural barrier to land transmission of disease-producing agents and has been aptly described as the cork in the bottle. FMD is the most used example: South America is generally infected and, as earlier mentioned, no country to the north has permitted the establishment of FMD.

As definitive plans for linking the Pan-American highway in the Darien Gap were drawn up in the early 1970s, concern over future disease introduction resulted in the formation of the Commission for the Prevention of Aftosa (COPFA) (formed to combat FMD) between the United States and Panama and the United States and Columbia. The reason is obvious, given the drive to open a modern highway through the Darien barrier.

Since formation, both commissions have worked to bolster defenses against disease spread should the highway be completed. On the Panamanian side, livestock-free zones were set up and a patrol force established; on the Columbian side, where some settlers and livestock were already present, a national park with controls over agricultural practices and homesteading was established in the western area.

The concern is not over the highway itself but over the anticipated development of previously undeveloped areas. In 1976 the codirectors of COPFA stated

> the position of COPFA is that the highway itself would not constitute any great danger for the entrance of foot and mouth disease from Columbia. It is very easy to establish quarantine and inspection stations to provide adequate control along the Highway, to restrict the entrance of hazardous materials and animals of the species susceptible of foot and mouth disease. The economic development resulting from the construction and completion of the Highway, are the factors that provide the greatest threat from animal diseases, including Aftosa. (Carrizo and Nelson 1976)

There are continuing arguments, pro and con, over the probable use or economic worth of a completed highway, considering the current political and military unrest in Central America. However, the real threat if the highway is finished is the opening of new areas, locally, for settlement and agricultural development across a barrier that historically has separated regions of differing disease status. If the highway is completed, a hemispheric approach to eliminating FMD will suddenly become of urgent self-interest to countries in the present island of North and Middle America.

# 3

# Economic and Cultural Perceptions

HUDSON (1983) PRESENTED the influence of disease control or eradication on the socioeconomic aspects of a society in terms of two self-perpetuating cycles: a negative cycle of a downward spiral of decreasing health levels creating steadily worsening socioeconomic conditions and, as a result of successful disease control efforts, a positive cycle of an upward spiral of increasing health levels that results in improvement of socioeconomic conditions.

The basic premises of the negative cycle are that diseased livestock are less productive than healthy animals, and lessened production results in lowered income and less animal protein and fiber for the producer and for society, thus lowering disposable income and further reducing expenditures for health. Deteriorating health conditions accelerate a downward spiral of health.

In relation to animal disease control and eradication, what kinds of people are we dealing with? If effective programs are to be developed, we must be aware of all who produce, consume, or otherwise relate to the animal population involved, inasmuch as the needs perceived by each segment will influence the overall acceptability of any proposal. In addition, the economic system within which the animals are produced, distributed, and consumed will markedly influence how services, including disease control activities, are developed.

Improvements in production efficiency require investment from some source. Disease control costs money. However, this may not be evident to many societies engaged in subsistence agriculture, using farming and husbandry procedures that produce little surplus beyond immediate local needs.

This situation appears to be changing in recent years with the revolution in world communications—including the transistor radio. This revolution brings to residents of areas with a tradition of subsistence agriculture knowledge of more efficient means of production plus increased aspirations for themselves and their families.

As production methods become more sophisticated, concern with efficiency (benefits vs. costs) increases, including recognition of disease control and eradication as an important facet of efficient production. Translating recognition into actions, however, requires investment. At the subsistence level the most elementary control measures may require outside help. Even in the so-called "developed" countries, large-scale disease control and eradication efforts are supported by public funds. In terms of public benefits such expenditures are justified politically and socially on the basis of the public value of improved production.

Bringing about such improvements by disease control or eradication programs requires recognizing that the programs themselves affect the social and economic conditions of society. In considering a program, the following factors should be studied:

1. What is the program's estimated benefit/cost ratio for the general public?

2. How is the disease perceived by the various groups that will be affected by the program?

3. What will the impact of the program be on these groups?

4. How will these groups react to the procedures required during the program?

5. How can all these perceptions and special interests be organized and united into coordinated support for a large-scale effort?

The costs of disease are many and varied. Death, though the least common, is the most dramatic; consequently, the use of public funds to control or eradicate disease has been concentrated on catastrophic diseases.

Well-informed producers may realize the hidden costs of less dramatic diseases as well as the associated costs of a disease control effort such as vaccines or drugs, veterinary services, construction of special facilities, and labor for treatment. These will not be understood by less knowledgeable owners. Without prior experience, no producer can appreciate large-scale program costs for such things as diagnostic surveys, quarantine administration, and disposal of infected flocks or herds. Public education in these areas is a critical part of early program development.

More difficult to assess, but just as real, is the psychological effect on individual owners, who, not knowing when or where the disease will strike next, feel uncertain about their means of livelihood. Perhaps even more damaging is development of a philosophy that disease is a natural phenomenon and losses are a normal, unalterable part of livestock production. It is virtually impossible to institute control or eradication programs in such an environment — where the losses are accepted as inevitable.

At both individual and national herd levels, loss of reputation due to the presence of a disease can be devastating. For decades diseases such as rinderpest, foot-and-mouth disease, trichinosis, and hog cholera have effectively halted much international movement of animal products. Today, what nation would consider purchasing pork products from a country where African swine fever is present?

Although consumerism has received much publicity in recent years, the adverse effects of buyer concern over animal health are not new. German consumers, fearful of trichinosis, were an important reason for the initiation of a mandatory meat inspection system in the United States at the turn of the century. Since 1969, when United States meat inspection laws were revised significantly, countries exporting meat and meat products to the United States have had to make many procedural changes in order to meet the requirements of U.S. consumers.

Because disease-producing agents usually reside in or on the affected animal, disease control or eradication efforts necessarily require actions involving the host animals. There are few exceptions to this rule, even for programs based on breaking the infectivity cycle by action against vector organisms such as ticks.

On-site testing, vaccination, inspection — all these require animal handling. Area quarantines restrict movement whether or not an individual producer within the area has an infected herd. Marketing restrictions, instituted as disease control measures, may reduce income by altering prices or reducing availability of markets.

In programs requiring compulsory disposition of infected individuals, flocks, or herds, owners seldom are compensated in full for their costs, even if indemnities are based on market value. Interruption of the income cycle, loss of years of breeding programs, idle pastures and facilities, and personal distress over removal of a cherished part of daily life and work are examples of direct program impact on such owners.

A localized area heavily affected by an eradication program may suffer disruption of many business operations. This disruption can include, in addition to the specific livestock or poultry operations concerned, other activities such as hatcheries, feeder-calf or feeder-pig suppliers outside the affected area, dairies, feed mills, livestock markets, processing plants, and trucking lines. Adverse reactions to these impacts can be expected even with the most careful thought and advanced planning. Successful programs hurt some people sometimes. Without effective prior attention to informing these people of what may be expected, and a strong effort to eliminate all unneeded procedural requirements, reaction by those affected may damage or halt the program.

Proper program planning includes time spent on anticipating when and where these adverse reactions will occur. Proper program execution requires monitoring program procedures to adjust, insofar as possible, those factors that are causing damage.

Talleyrand, the French diplomat and statesman of the early nineteenth century, is reported to have said, in effect, that every negotiator should spend 10 minutes of every working hour trying to see the question at issue through the eyes of the adversary. This is a good working precept for those engaged in administering animal health programs, which usually are designed to benefit many who have little involvement in the program by imposing upon a few who often are involved far beyond their desires.

This sensitivity must be extended beyond the obvious cause and effect of a program. Health professionals perceive specific program procedures and requirements in terms of what they will do for the programs. Persons affected by these procedures may perceive them in very different terms.

When the United States embarked on a program to eradicate hog cholera, it was "self-evident" to animal health officials that an early need was a quarantine system for infected herds. Yet market research conducted for hog cholera biologics producers at that time showed that fewer than 2% of the swine producers believed that quarantining was an important protective measure (Elrick and Lovidge 1961). It is disheartening to hear an industry spokesman claim that more producers will be put out of business by the eradication program than by the disease.

## Economic Perceptions

It is easy to see how producers can be convinced that participation in a disease control or eradication program is beneficial if their animals are dying and the program will cost them little or nothing. However, programs are not that simple or clear cut, and those whose herds are affected by the disease and will benefit from the program will generally experience some losses from the program as well. This has led producers to be suspicious of veterinarians who talk glibly of an easy route to disease-free herds. Programs that involve testing to detect infected animals often also involve slaughtering these animals, with the owner being compensated at less than the perceived or actual value of the animals. Unfortunately, in many instances, this aspect of the program is not fully explained to producers in terms they understand, including how this will protect their herds in the future. A producer in this situation often becomes bitter and uncooperative and fails to present all his animals for testing. Another reason for lack of cooperation is that in countries where vaccines are administered free of charge, such as for rinderpest, the number of reported livestock vaccinated will be recorded. This number, in turn, may be used to determine the amount of tax owed by the producer—an additional use of information beyond determining the number of vaccine doses needed in future vaccination rounds. Underreporting then ensues in order to avoid full taxation, which results in insufficient vaccination levels. In both examples the level of producer participation needed for program success becomes inadequate.

To initiate a disease program without first carefully assessing the wants of consumers and producers alike is to invite failure. Generally, livestock owners are unwilling to spend money on disease control or eradication unless they are convinced the disease costs more money than does the proposed program. If they do not perceive a net economic loss, they will not give high priority to committing their cooperation and resources to the program. Consumers, whose desires usually are communicated through the political process, feel strongly about protecting the safety and quality of their food supply. They see this as more important than food producers' concerns over adverse effects of control programs.

## Cultural Perceptions

Culture can be thought of as the sum of the attitudes and expectations of a particular society. While these are learned by individuals growing up in that society, the end result is a pattern of thought or action that is widely character-istic for the group—these can change for a society over time. Instant long-distance communication, common today in most societies of any size, has produced many cultural changes; yet less than two centuries ago no society had such abilities. In smaller groups, cultural change can be particularly rapid and sweeping following exposure to new influences or technology from a previously foreign society.

Examples of this latter situation can be found in any part of the world where previously distinct cultures came together. The illustrations discussed below are from North America.

Horses disappeared from the Western Hemisphere in prehistoric times, not to reappear until the Spanish arrived in the sixteenth century. At that time the western plains of North America were peopled by tribal societies whose culture, which had developed in the environment over thousands of years, was based on the limits of human physical capability. Then, as a result of Spanish explorations northward, these tribal groups began to acquire horses. In the early nineteenth century when northern Europeans reached the western plains, they found native societies whose culture was centered on the use of horses for hunting, transport, warfare, and measurement of wealth. In less than three centuries a new way of life had been developed.

In the Arctic, indigenous societies with a record of survival over many centuries in an extremely harsh environment with no metal, little wood, and little food supply directly from plants, have been exposed in the nineteenth and twentieth centuries to cultures with metals, foods derived from agri-cultural effort, and mechanical sophistication beyond anything they previously knew. Now, in most Arctic areas of Canada and Alaska, snowmobiles have largely replaced dog teams, bone tools are no longer essential, and outboard motors and guns have revolutionized hunting. The availability of quantities of oil and new technology has permitted rapid, worldwide cultural change, which is spectacularly illustrated by the revolution in life-styles in the last 100 years. Presumably, in these situations, the original culture was altered because most members believed that adherence to custom was foolish in view of the convenience and luxury to be gained by abandoning the past. But deeply rooted cultural practices or religious beliefs may delay or deter adoption of change. There are still certain groups, because of strong religious convictions, that avoid the gasoline engine. For similar reasons, the emergence of a swine industry in Semitic cultures is unlikely.

Two prime concepts relative to disease control can be drawn from this. One is that cultural characteristics will influence how a particular group will evaluate the need for, or procedures used in, a disease control program. Therefore, it is important to learn cultural patterns of affected groups while developing a program. This need for assistance from those familiar with the cultures or subcultures affected is particularly strong when an international program is under consideration. For example, during the international smallpox eradication campaign, the administrators of the program in some West African countries had to reckon with a smallpox cult that related the disease to the gods, including the practice of virus inoculation (Foege et al. 1975). Dealing successfully with this subculture obviously presented challenges different from those in societies without this religious orientation.

The other concept to be kept in mind is that cultural attitudes can change, and specific attitudes can change rapidly, even during the course of a single program. The challenge for health professionals is to utilize, as necessary, this ability for cultural change to maintain program progress. Such changes may be influenced but cannot be imposed. They must be allowed to develop at a pace consistent with the perceptions of the affected group. Therefore, it is these perceptions that are the key factor in bringing about change. Demands from outside the affected group that a change must be made are usually ineffectual and can be calamitous.

An example can be given from the hog cholera eradication program in the United States. When the program started in 1962, the swine industry had a cultural attitude, based on experience, that centered on vaccination as the primary means of control. This situation had existed for half a century and few other control measures were used. Although vaccination had become the largest single expense associated with the disease, any attempt by program administrators to quickly remove vaccines, even if sound, would have been unacceptable to an industry that thought in terms of little other than vaccination when thinking of hog cholera control. Changes in public attitudes regarding the disease, including vaccination, came about rapidly during the program as other disease prevention techniques were adopted and as more information on the risks as well as the value of vaccination was accumulated and disseminated. By 1967, only 5 years later, an advisory panel recommended that hog cholera vaccination be phased out. The plan received majority support that enabled such action by 1970 — a step that would have been impossible in 1962.

Organized public disease control and eradication programs are political in nature, a fact of life that must be instilled in anyone devoting a career to such programs. As disease control and eradication cannot be expected to be of sufficient importance to override all other political considerations, health programs must be compatible with political realities. This calls for ingenuity and a recognition that most destinations can be reached by more than one road. The key is to use open roads and not waste time on closed routes.

Disposition of infected herds illustrates the varied approaches utilized under varying political systems. One system is based on state ownership of property to the extent that there is no significant private ownership of agricultural resources, including livestock or poultry. Since there is no question of private ownership to deal with, no individual rights are involved, and, theoretically at least, condemnation can be initiated at any time the state wishes.

Another political system, while based on private ownership of property, allows condemnation of private property but does not require or support compensation to owners whose property is condemned. The owner absorbs the total loss. In this circumstance, early imposition of compulsory herd disposition, when infection rates are high, would arouse strong opposition. Therefore, a program under this system must be designed to delay herd condemnation until infection is rare, and the isolated and unfortunate owner of such a herd stands alone.

A third political system, also based on private ownership of property, permits the state to condemn private property but requires that owners be compensated. In this situation, it is possible to move more rapidly into elimination of infected herds and shorten the length of the program. A necessary restraint under this system, however, is not to move into payment of compensation without a good knowledge of how much infection remains. Moving too soon results in indemnity costs exceeding original predictions, placing the program in political jeopardy because of these unanticipated costs.

These are not hypothetical situations. All these political systems exist in countries pursuing animal disease control and eradication programs. Each situation requires a different approach, yet it is not a question of which is best; that is irrelevant. The reality is that a program operationally based on one political system cannot be expected to function if transplanted into a different political system with a different structure.

Sensitivity to societal differences is important, not only in international programs, but within a country. No nations of significant size have uniform societies made up of people and groups that see everything from the same viewpoint.

# 4

# Historical Precepts

STUDIES OF ANCIENT HUMAN SOCIETIES show that efforts to prevent or alleviate illness go back many thousands of years.

Six hundred centuries ago, in a highlands cave in what is now Iraq, a band of Neanderthal people decorated a grave with a variety of flowering plants. Studies of pollen remains show that several of these plants continued to be used locally as herbal medicines until recent times (Leakey and Lewin 1977).

In Neolithic times, skulls were being trepanned, possibly to release demons possessing the mind of the patient. The bone fragment removed appears to have been valuable as an amulet — so much so that demand exceeded supply and counterfeits made from animal bone have been found (Smithcors 1957), demonstrating that sharp business practices also have a long history.

Chapters 13 and 14 of the Old Testament book of Leviticus contain a detailed clinical guide for the diagnosis of leprosy, the segregation of people found to be infected, and rituals for the cleansing of garments and dwellings. We may no longer accept many of the procedures prescribed, but it is evident they were based on an understanding of the process of contagion.

More than two thousand years ago during the Vedic civilization in what is now India, a humanitarian king set up hundreds of veterinary hospitals, staffed by state paid practitioners, where many species were studied and treated and diseases described that seem to include rinderpest, anthrax, and piroplasmosis. By A.D. 500 the successors of that culture apparently were aware of the relationship of mosquitoes to malaria and of rats to human plague, were splinting fractures, performing Caesarian sections, and operating on urinary calculi (Smithcors 1957).

These early efforts toward health protection, and most medicine in the centuries since, were based on conclusions gained empirically as opposed to what we would now call scientific knowledge.

> The goal of Aristotelean science was to explain *why* things happen. Modern science was born when Galileo began to explain *how* things happen and thus originated the method of controlled experiment which now forms the basis of scientific investigation. (Barnett 1948)

The Aristotelean belief that reality could be found by reasoning from a base of self-evident truths did at times lead in the right direction, as illustrated by some of the preceding examples. However, as it depended on "self-evident" facts rather than those established by experiment, it could also lead down paths now regarded as fanciful, such as the belief that persisted into relatively modern times that life forms could arise through spontaneous generation.

Yet, in spite of the immense leaps in scientific medical knowledge in the past few generations, credit for the basic tenets of large-scale disease control and eradication must go to earlier individuals who observed illness, concluded what might be happening, and developed the principles of search, quarantine, and destroy, which today remain the foundation for attacking disease. Successful programs are still dependent on rigorous application of these precepts, and failures are due to the inability or unwillingness to do so.

## The Rise of Modern Medicine

With the beginning of the seventeenth century and the experimental approach of Galileo, and in spite of pervasive superstitions regarding disease, modern medical science began to emerge. Acceptance of new ideas was no easier then than it is today. In the 1600s Francisco Redi showed that maggots were not spontaneously generated when he eliminated their development by screening meat with fine gauze. But it was not until 1877 that John Tyndall ended the argument by originating a system of fractional sterilization that could eliminate resistant spores, whose unexplained presence had led die-hard proponents to continue insisting that spontaneous generation was still a valid source of living microorganisms (Merchant 1940).

Starting with the Renaissance, isolated applications of the experimental approach to the study of disease led to multiple discoveries during the nineteenth century. In 1876 this culminated in conclusive proof of the germ theory through Koch's work on anthrax. Pasteur's studies of anthrax and rabies established the attenuation of bacteria and viruses as a basis for immunization. Lister demonstrated that the use of dressings treated with carbolic acid following surgery would reduce infection. Across the Atlantic, Smith, Kilbourne, and Curtice first identified intracellular protozoa as a cause of illness and demonstrated transmission through an intermediate host. These veterinarians, working with the piroplasm causing tick fever in cattle, opened the way for action against typhus, yellow fever, malaria, and other vector-borne diseases.

During the eighteenth century rinderpest (cattle plague), a follower of military campaigns, and the need to import live cattle in the days before mechanical refrigeration continued to rise and fall across Europe. This and other animal disease problems led to the establishment of the Lyons and Alfort veterinary schools in France in the 1760s. By 1800 there were 20 veterinary schools in 12 European countries.

Smithcors (1957) assembled a review of rinderpest in Europe during the

1700s that illustrates both the early recognition of sound disease control principles and the consequences of failure to follow these principles. He estimates that over 200 million cattle died from rinderpest in western Europe between 1711 and 1769. Most outbreaks received little constructive attention, and a variety of treatments were touted as the way to handle the disease. One popular treatment on the continent was the administration of several dozen bottles of wine per cow—costly, but perhaps of some anaesthetic value to the animal in its final days.

However, in a 1713 outbreak in Italy, Giovanni Lancisi, physician to Pope Clement XI, stated that rinderpest was contagious and recommended the following program, with severe punishment for those who did not comply.

1. Sick animals must be separated from well animals.

2. Infected animals must be slaughtered immediately by stunning (no bleeding) and the carcasses buried in a deep pit.

3. Any ox or dog that gains entry to the area must be destroyed.

4. No attempt must be made to treat sick animals.

5. Healthy animals should be removed from infected pastures.

6. Feeding and veterinary equipment should be cleaned with quicklime and handlers' clothes fumigated.

The outbreak in the Rome area was eliminated in 9 months but continued in other areas for several years. Lancisi's principles were ignored in later outbreaks in Italy in 1730, 1735, and again in 1744, and the disease was left to run its course.

In France, where from 1710 to 1714 rinderpest was reported as killing 50% of the cattle population, Lancisi's program was finally used in 1774 after several additional cycles of the disease.

During the same period that Lancisi was working in Rome, cattle imported from Holland caused an outbreak in the London area. In 1714 Thomas Bates, surgeon to the crown, was appointed to investigate; he subsequently developed similar proposals.

1. All cattle in affected herds should be killed.

2. Barns should be washed and fumigated and vacated for 3 months.

3. Handlers of the infected herd should be prevented from contacting other cattle.

4. The herd should be divided into small groups for pasture.

The resulting control program for this outbreak also saw the initial use of indemnities, paid as a bounty from the royal treasury. The bounty was set at about 2 pounds for a cow sick less than 24 hours, and ½ pound if the owner delayed reporting—a most effective way to encourage prompt reporting, and one that unfortunately has been too often ignored in programs since that time.

Unfortunately, a 1745 introduction of rinderpest, which Parliament tried to handle without vigorous application of Bates's precepts, ran on until 1756, with a loss of several hundred thousand cattle. Finally, following another outbreak in 1769, his program was again used.

Rinderpest, contagious bovine pleuropneumonia (CBPP), and other damaging animal diseases, including foot-and-mouth disease (FMD) in England in 1839, led to increasingly stringent national regulatory acts during the nineteenth century and the establishment of a Board of Agriculture in 1887. This board had a veterinary department and responsibility for enforcing the Contagious Diseases of Animals Acts. A slaughter policy was extended to CBPP and FMD in the 1890s.

The continued presence of rinderpest on the European continent led to an international conference in Vienna in 1872 at which it was agreed that member countries would be immediately notified of any outbreaks and informed of the progress of efforts to eliminate such outbreaks; this was the beginning for international animal disease reporting systems. The diseases CBPP and FMD continued as problems in Europe, and national veterinary departments came into being to combat these problems and other endemic diseases. Cycles of rinderpest ceased in Europe in 1880 except for a brief introduction in Belgium in 1920. Although CBPP entered briefly from the East in World War I, it was similarly controlled and finally eliminated from western Europe. By the end of the 1800s after almost two centuries of fitful application of sound control and eradication principles, veterinary schools and national animal health agencies knew what had to be done — at least for contagions that could be diagnosed by experienced clinicians and were transmitted directly.

The development of successful disease control principles in England and western Europe also had wider influence. Politically, the nineteenth century was a period when these countries had much of the world under colonial status. The influence of Britain was particularly important, since that country became the most widespread empire in world history. British laws and concepts regarding animal diseases were transplanted to other regions, including their African colonies, Australia, and Canada, establishing traditions and practices that have persisted.

Another important nineteenth-century development influencing international animal disease control was the initiation of artificial refrigeration. From 1774 on, commercial shipment of live cattle had been responsible for the introduction of rinderpest into 33 countries previously free of the disease (USLSA 1964). Refrigerated shipping was first used to transport chilled beef from the United States to Great Britain in 1875; it was soon expanded to move carcass meat from Australia and New Zealand to Great Britain and Europe. Refrigerated ships and railway cars reduced the need to import live animals for slaughter and greatly reduced the risk of disease introduction.

It is useful to keep in mind, however, that clear thinkers such as Lancisi and Bates, without the advantage of modern scientific medical supports, developed programs to eliminate disease that contain the basic principles still required to do the work successfully. With these principles it was possible to eliminate rinderpest and CBPP even before the causative agents were known. The virus causing rinderpest was not identified until 1902, 22 years after endemic rinderpest had been eliminated from Europe; CBPP was eradicated from the United States before the agent had been identified.

The many failures to contain and remove outbreaks of these diseases in the eighteenth and nineteenth centuries resulted from the lack of application of known principles rather than from the lack of knowledge. In spite of the current wealth of medical knowledge, program failures are still usually due to a lack of courage in promptly and vigorously following measures to locate the disease, contain it from further spread, destroy the foci of infection, and clean up contaminated facilities.

## Colonization of North America

On the North American continent, Mexico was originally the northern anchor of the Spanish colonial empire that stretched south to the tip of South America. Early Spanish emphasis was on treasure rather than on agriculture. The large livestock enterprises that later developed in Spanish North America did not, in early years, directly contact or influence the type of livestock development in the rest of the continent.

The northern territories of the continent were under the early influence of the French. The French explorers developed a relatively enlightened attitude toward the indigenous tribes, which laid the foundation for an enormously profitable fur trade. Commercial agriculture, including livestock production, was not essential for a profitable colonial venture in New France.

Between the French to the north and the Spanish to the south, and relatively untouched by European exploitation during the 1500s, lay the Atlantic coast of what is now the United States. Following defeat of the Spanish Armada in 1588, England began to expand as a world power, and colonists began arriving along this coast in the early 1600s. By the early 1700s, expansion of the colonies was perceived by the French as an encroachment on their fur-trading territory. The French and English engaged in a series of military campaigns, which resulted in the transfer of New France to the British crown. Increased immigration, primarily by the English, led to the further development of the new land, with a gradual increased emphasis on agriculture and livestock production.

Although earlier peoples had preceded the Europeans by thousands of years and had developed numerous societies from the Arctic to Tierra del Fuego, they had migrated from the Old World long before the domestication of plants and animals. The indigenous American cultures independently dis-

OLSON LIBRARY
NORTHERN MICHIGAN UNIVERSITY
MARQUETTE, MICHIGAN   49855

covered cultivation of plants, but with the exception of the turkey, the guinea pig, and the llama-alpaca family, they did not domesticate any American animal species for food or draft.

Cattle were introduced when Columbus returned to the Caribbean in 1493. By the time of the Plymouth colony in Massachusetts in 1620, domestic livestock of various species were a part of settlements from Nova Scotia in the north through the Spanish colonies in South America.

Human diseases brought by the Europeans found susceptible hosts in the native peoples of the Americas, and many of these societies were decimated by disease. The diseases of imported European livestock had no comparable population to attack. Livestock introductions were infrequent, small in numbers, and there was little opportunity for further spread of the diseases that did arrive. Immigrant livestock apparently did not encounter significant new diseases upon arrival; consequently, animal diseases were seldom mentioned in records of the colonial period in North America.

In Europe, with long land borders between nations, restricting the movement of animal disease has always been difficult. Before the relatively recent demonstration of the germ theory of disease as fact, the idea of unseen transmissible life forms as the cause of illness was unknown. Although a few early observers had noted that quarantine measures were valuable in disease prevention, the fact that less dramatic infections could move across borders within apparently healthy individuals was still centuries away from discovery.

Even though the natural quarantine protection afforded the New World was fortuitous rather than planned, it operated well as long as livestock shipments from Europe were few in number and European enclaves in the Americas were small and isolated. Acute illness took its toll during the long voyage from the Old World. The more chronic and less obvious illnesses, if they survived the trip, had no easy way to spread since the European settlements had limited contact with one another. Rinderpest, for example, never reached the Americas in the colonial period even though the disease was endemic in Europe. Foot-and-mouth disease, apparently present in Europe since at least 1514 (Callis and Shahan 1970), did not reach North America until 1870.

These unplanned barriers, which apparently provided reasonably good protection well into the eighteenth century, began to break down as ocean traffic between Europe and North America increased and the colonies expanded and became less isolated. As the numbers of imported livestock grew, so did the probability of new infections gaining entry. As communication and trade increased between the colonies, so did the opportunities for spread of such infections.

# 5

## The Americas: Past Problems and Some Solutions

### United States

Toward the end of the eighteenth century the United States, with a growing and diversifying livestock population, began to experience widespread animal disease problems that rapidly grew in magnitude and variety.

A forecast of things to come was provided by the spread of what came to be known as cattle tick fever (bovine piroplasmosis), which became a major disease problem in the eastern United States by the late 1700s. Presumably entering from Spanish territories to the south, cattle tick fever was so prevalent by 1795 that North Carolina prohibited entry of cattle from South Carolina and Georgia from March to November, when the risk to local cattle was greatest. An outbreak in eastern Pennsylvania in the summer of 1796, attributed to cattle from South Carolina, was reported in a Philadelphia agricultural journal with the observation that it was a mystery why the southern cattle themselves showed no illness (Bierer [1939] 1974).

In the nineteenth century, with the rapid expansion of transportation, population, and territory, animal diseases grew to alarming proportions. Bierer's inventory of reports of significant maladies from 1800 to 1884 includes the following diseases:

1. "Mad itch": By the 1820s, infection was reported from Pennsylvania to Missouri.
2. Hog cholera: This disease progressed from the Ohio River basin in the 1830s to the East Coast and Louisiana by 1866.
3. Anthrax: Presence of the disease was reported from Pennsylvania to Kentucky by 1833.
4. Bovine abortion: Reported from Pennsylvania in 1843, the disease was

27

troublesome in the East and Midwest by 1868. Dairymen feared that comment on the disease might start public concern.

5. Contagious bovine pleuropneumonia: This disease was introduced in 1843 and spread west to Missouri by 1884.

6. "Dreadful mortality": This disease of horses (probably equine encephalomyelitis) was reported from Massachusetts to St. Louis by 1846.

7. Cattle tick fever: This disease was causing heavy losses from Massachusetts to Kansas and along drovers' routes from Texas to Illinois as early as 1854.

8. Foot-and-mouth disease: The first report of this disease was in New England in 1870.

9. Equine influenza: This disease spread nationwide from 1872 to 1875, causing interruptions in transport, farming, and lumbering.

10. Fowl cholera: In 1877 heavy losses from this disease were reported from Ohio to Texas.

11. "Enzootic" ergotism: This disease, reported in cattle in Kansas in 1884, was first thought to be virulent foot-and-mouth disease. It caused unsteady cattle prices.

Systematic attention to animal disease losses began after the Department of Agriculture was established in 1862. The work of J. R. Dodge, statistician of the department, resulted in a flow of reports on the large losses being experienced. In a country where much of the income and most of the employment was dependent on agriculture, these reports aroused wide concern. Public demands for action made animal disease losses a matter of political importance.

At the end of the Civil War there was no organized system for dealing with animal diseases. Although a veterinary school had been established in Mexico in 1853 and Canada had established state supported veterinary training in 1862, veterinary education in the United States was limited to private schools, operated for profit.

In 1868 the Commissioner of Agriculture reported that huge disease losses in farm animals called for government action and the formation of veterinary colleges to educate practitioners. The first publicly supported school was started at Iowa State College in 1871.

In 1869 and 1870 the commissioner recommended that a division of veterinary surgery be established in the Department of Agriculture. In 1880 another commissioner concluded that "the ravages of disease in this country among various animals of economic value have become alarmingly great. . . . In no way can the remedy be made so effective as through a suitable organized division of veterinary science attached to this Department" (USDA 1880).

Through the years animal health continued to deteriorate. In 1879 Great Britain removed the United States from its import list due to contagious bovine pleuropneumonia (CBPP), which had been present for over 40 years without a national effort to eliminate the problem. By 1883 European countries were banning U.S. pork because of the risk to consumers from trichinosis. Hog cholera, cattle tick fever, and abortion disease (presumably brucellosis) continued to spread. Finally, in 1883 as a result of continued requests of the Commissioner of Agriculture, an experiment station was established to investigate contagious diseases of domestic animals.

Political pressure finally caused Congress to act, and in 1884 the Bureau of Animal Industry (BAI) was created as part of the Department of Agriculture. The BAI was to be headed by a competent veterinary surgeon and was charged with investigating the condition of domestic animals, the causes of their diseases, and the means for cure and prevention. To meet this large responsibility the Commissioner of Agriculture was authorized to employ a force sufficient for this purpose, but not to exceed 20 persons at any time.

The bureau promptly initiated an eradication program against CBPP, extensive studies of hog cholera, and the investigation of cattle tick fever. By 1892 CBPP had been eradicated. The decades of national confusion and inactivity regarding animal disease had been replaced by an organized national presence actively pursuing research, prevention, and eradication.

While the BAI quickly gained a national and international reputation in veterinary science and preventive medicine, there were many problems and errors. However, one of the strengths of the organization was the ability to recognize and correct deficiencies and work to successful conclusions, many of which today appear to be automatic.

The following eradication programs for three significant livestock diseases eliminated from the United States illustrate some of the pitfalls in attitudes and actions that must be watched for in animal health work.

**CONTAGIOUS BOVINE PLEUROPNEUMONIA.** Although endemic in the New York City area since 1843, CBPP entered Massachusetts in 1859 via imported Dutch cattle, causing great concern in surrounding areas. A special report on the disease was presented in the 1860 census (Eighth Census) of the United States (Bierer [1939] 1974). In special session, the Massachusetts legislature appropriated $1 million and adopted a program of mandatory reporting, isolation, and branding of infected and exposed cattle; compensation for maintenance and destruction with indemnities as ordered; and control of cattle movement. These measures arrested the disease in Massachusetts. Unfortunately, other states did not follow suit and CBPP continued to spread with no accurate determination of prevalence.

The first national animal disease eradication campaign in the United States (under the BAI) started in 1884. By then CBPP had spread west to Missouri. In spite of the demonstrated success of the techniques used in Massachusetts 25 years previously, the national program was hampered initially by shortages of indemnity funds and lack of sufficient authority to condemn exposed cattle. Later legislation corrected these deficiencies and the infected zones were rapidly reduced. Final eradication occurred in 1892, which enabled the Secretary of Agriculture to report to the President that "in spite of all obstacles, often times of unjust criticism, and of virulent opposition in some sectors, our officers have succeeded in doing what at the onset was declared by many as an impossible achievement." The secretary also noted that $1.5 million spent on the program in the United States was less than that spent for indemnity alone in Great Britain from 1883 to 1890, and Great Britain had not yet succeeded in eradicating the disease (USDA 1892).

**FOOT-AND-MOUTH DISEASE.** The course of eradication of foot-and-mouth disease (FMD) in the United States has not always demonstrated the necessity or the practice of rapid and vigorous intervention by organized veterinary medicine. Although the disease has never become established and there has been a stamping-out policy since 1902, no action was taken in some early cases; inertia occurred later.

There were three introductions of disease recorded as FMD in the nineteenth century. In the winter of 1870, the disease spread south from Canada into New England. The relative isolation and lack of movement of livestock did not encourage perpetuation; the disease died out before the warm months. In the early 1880s, two individual herd infections died out without spreading (Diamant 1978).

Outbreaks in 1902 and 1908 were different. In November 1902 FMD was reported from Massachusetts through Vermont, New Hampshire, and into Rhode Island. Disagreement by Massachusetts authorities on how to handle the problem led Congress, in early 1903, to give the BAI authority to override the states in controlling international and interstate transportation of livestock; eradication was achieved within the year.

In November 1908 FMD was found in Pennsylvania. By the end of the month Pennsylvania, New York, Michigan, and Maryland were under quarantine. The eradication effort was rapidly concluded within 6 months. In contrast to nineteenth-century introductions from imported animals, investigation of the 1908 outbreak implicated contaminated smallpox virus imported for vaccine production. The virus was sent to a biologics firm in Detroit and used to infect calves inoculated for human vaccine production; FMD spread to eastern states when the calves moved through the Detroit stockyards (Bierer [1939] 1974). The investigation also concluded that the origin of the 1902 outbreak had been similar.

The BAI and the states, after demonstrating in 1902 and 1908 their ability to quickly eradicate FMD even after it had spread into several states, were not as successful a few years later. In 1914 FMD started in Michigan and eventually spread to 22 states and Puerto Rico, becoming the largest outbreak in U.S. history. This outbreak (1914–1916) demonstrated the unfortunate results of a lack of attention in early weeks and months and illustrated what can happen when a potentially explosive disease is initially approached on a casual basis.

In August 1914 sick hogs were noted on a farm in southwest Michigan. When other farms became affected, state authorities were called in, but the source could not be located. A month later a BAI veterinarian investigated the problem at the request of the state; FMD was suspected, but the report cited necrotic stomatitis, not FMD.

Within the second month, the sickness had spread to six more farms, with a clinical picture implicating FMD. A BAI veterinarian made a clinical diagnosis of FMD, which was confirmed by animal inoculation tests. Quarantines were finally applied in Michigan and Indiana 11 weeks after the disease had first appeared. However, by this time FMD had spread beyond the quarantined area, and 20 states were affected by the end of November, causing cancellation of the annual meeting of the American Veterinary Medical Association to free the profession to fight the disease. Eradication required a massive effort throughout 1915 into 1916. Final quarantines were not removed until June 1916, almost 2 years after the initial outbreak (Bierer [1939] 1974; Smithcors 1963).

Studies of animal movements during the early weeks of this outbreak show the multiplication of exposure that can develop from a dilatory approach to a disease emergency. During the 11 weeks from the initial illness to the first quarantines, milk from an infected dairy farm was sent to a local creamery, from which skimmed milk used to feed livestock produced further outbreaks. Two weeks before the first quarantine action, cattle, sheep, and swine from the infected area were shipped to the Chicago stockyards, and from there the disease continued to spread (Smithcors 1963).

Such uncontrolled widening of exposure before regulatory action was taken resulted in public uncertainty, political vacillation, and attempts to avoid economic loss. Owners rushed animals to market when they saw or anticipated the onset of disease, which only resulted in additional exposure.

The initial source of FMD in this outbreak was not specifically identified, although the Michigan hogs where the disease first appeared were reported to have been fed trimmings and offal from a slaughterhouse handling foreign meats (Mohler 1924). Therefore in 1914, as in 1902 and 1908, the greatest risk from FMD appeared to no longer be imported animals themselves, but products and by-products of animal origin. In addition, although the actual stamping-out program was a demonstration of well-organized disease eradication, actions in the initial weeks were not up to standard.

After this experience the BAI set up standby plans and policies to ensure prompt reaction should there be future introductions. Predesignated field veterinarians were equipped in advance to go immediately to the scene of a suspicious report. Also, policies to ensure prompt diagnostic decisions and regulatory responses were prepared, as well as standby plans for a broad public education program. These were tested when FMD struck in California and Texas in 1924 and again in California in 1929.

Suspected FMD was reported in the San Francisco area in February 1924 in hogs fed garbage from the Mare Island Navy Yard. Initial diagnosis and quarantining was rapid and within a week the first infected herd had been destroyed and buried. It took 20 months to stamp out this outbreak, but the bulk of the time was required to eliminate FMD from the deer herds in a national forest infected when summer grazing grounds received infected stock.

In 1924 a separate outbreak occurred in the Houston area; this was eliminated in 30 days. In 1929 in the Los Angeles area, FMD appeared in swine that had been fed garbage from a ship carrying South American meat. Reaction to the outbreak was quick and the infected herds were eliminated in 60 days.

With six outbreaks of FMD from 1902 through 1929, regulations to prevent introduction of the disease had proved inadequate. The BAI and the states demonstrated they could handle outbreaks that did occur, but it was evident that the same capability did not extend to preventing disease in the first place.

The result was amendments to the Tariff Act of 1930, which prohibited entry of all domestic cloven-hoofed animals and fresh, chilled, or frozen meat from such animals from countries infected with FMD or rinderpest. With this action Congress not only removed USDA discretional authority over such entries, but also expressed an import philosophy of avoiding any possibility of disease rather than one of merely trying to lower the probability of doing so. Since 1930 USDA requirements have been aimed at removing any risk and are regarded as severe by importers and many other countries. With this policy, however, the United States has remained free of FMD for over half a century. Whether this is due to fortunate coincidence or cause and effect may be debatable, but the results are dramatically improved over earlier years.

**VESICULAR EXANTHEMA OF SWINE.** In disease eradication, acts of omission are usually more costly than acts of commission. The history of vesicular exanthema of swine (VES) illustrates the cost of delayed action and that later events may require revision of the initial policy.

In 1932 in Southern California, a vesicular disease appeared in garbage-fed swine. Initially diagnosed as FMD, the herd was destroyed, with the BAI participating with the state. Another outbreak occurred in swine the next year. Studies determined that the agent was not FMD virus but a previously unidentified virus producing symptoms in swine clinically indistinguishable from FMD (Traum 1934). The new disease was called vesicular exanthema of swine.

With FMD ruled out, the BAI apparently decided that continuing a cooperative eradication campaign would be beyond its scope of authority, so California was left to handle the problem. For the next 20 years VES outbreaks continued in California, confined almost exclusively to garbage-feeding operations. It became evident to California officials that the usual method of spread was feeding swine uncooked garbage. However, neither California on the state level, nor the BAI on the national level, adopted garbage-cooking requirements, even though Canada had done so as early as 1916 as part of its hog cholera eradication effort. California expended much effort studying the disease and trying to find effective means, other than garbage cooking, to contain the infection.

The federal attitude changed in 1952 when VES rapidly spread east from California and infected other parts of the country. The livestock industry, the states, and the federal government decided that the national risk of masking an introduction of FMD would be too great if VES was allowed to become endemic throughout the United States. A federal-state eradication campaign eliminated VES by 1956; eradication was declared in 1959. As with the FMD eradication effort in 1914–1916, the USDA and the states had shown the ability to stamp out disease, but only after early inaction had led to widespread infection before the campaign was initiated.

**FEDERAL-STATE COOPERATION.** The BAI was dissolved in 1953. During the 70 years between 1884 and 1953 the BAI was the single most important influence in initiating and promoting large, organized animal disease control and eradication programs.

While the preceding section emphasized some of the pitfalls to be watched for in campaigns against animal disease, using selected programs as examples, the impact of the variety and quality of the work done by this agency is still evident. Among the most important achievements was the initiation and perpetuation of a system of cooperative federal and state programs that retains individual state authority and yet enables sufficient uniformity to reach a single nationwide goal.

In 1886 an initial step in the first animal disease eradication program in the United States was a cooperative memorandum of understanding executed between the BAI and the state of Illinois. The pattern of this joint agreement, which outlined the essential features of a CBPP eradication program and how each party would function under the agreement, was followed in other states in the CBPP campaign and has continued in all federal-state programs since that time.

The nature of large-scale animal health programs in the United States cannot be understood without an understanding of why such an arrangement is necessary and how the cooperative process has functioned. In size and complexity, it is a system unique to the United States and results from the division of the power to regulate under the U.S. Constitution.

The Constitution reserves certain police powers for the federal government. The states have the authority and responsibility for administering those powers not reserved for the federal government. As far as animal health is concerned, states generally hold authority for action within their borders, and the federal government holds authority for regulating interstate and international matters, those that can affect the entire nation. There are certain emergency circumstances in which the federal government assumes authority within a state; however, the bulk of animal health program activity is under state control, including reporting of disease, quarantining, compulsory condemnation of animals and materials, and controlling animal movement within a state.

The cooperative agreement between the BAI and Illinois not only was a way for the two parties to operate under a constitutionally divided authority structure, but also it provided a means, through similar agreements with other states, for general uniformity in program goals and operation. Such agreements outline not only a national program philosophy but also provide some assurance that other states in the program will operate under the same general rules.

Given the variety of specific diseases and animal production systems in the 50 states with many subdivisions of authority, it is difficult and time consuming to arrive at a reasonable consensus among all these jurisdictions. To meet this challenge, the states and the BAI came together before the end of the nineteenth century in a national consultative organization to debate animal health questions and try to arrive at mutually acceptable policies.

Since 1897 this group, known as the United States Animal Health Association, has been the deliberative body for animal health program work in the United States. Without authority or means of funding programs, the organization has provided a successful means for building a common approach to animal health work of national consequence. The association is made up of the chief animal health officials of each state and the federal government, plus members of the livestock industry and veterinary research and education. The standing committees of this organization discuss varying points of view on technical and operational questions, monitor the progress of programs in operation, and recommend areas for change.

There are advantages to such a system beyond the need to cope with division of authority. The United States is a country of 3.6 million square miles, including almost every type of climate and geography in which livestock and poultry can be raised. Animal husbandry and marketing practices vary widely, as do diseases and their manifestations. No single national government authority could be expected to know or to take into proper account all these differences in designing and operating programs. Each state, however, is close to its own situation and can argue for programs structured to its needs. From these arguments a general framework, with opportunity for individual variation, usually evolves. Although quick decisions for initial action or program changes are infrequent under the system, the need for federal and state consultation helps to prevent a single national agency from making important errors of judgment.

A further advantage to the nation is the opportunity for pilot program action; new and untried programs can be tested cooperatively. A relatively small field effort can test what will or will not be effective under field conditions on a statewide basis, another means of avoiding errors on a national scale.

Another important value under a nonauthoritarian political system is that once a program is generally agreed upon by the state and federal animal health authorities, along with livestock industry representatives, broad political support for carrying out the work is much stronger than if a single federal group had to convince not only Congress but also each state government.

However, even the best cooperation among animal health authorities cannot be expected to offset the delay between technical ability to attack a problem and the public will to do so, often evident in a democratic political system. Such delays have been frequent in the history of animal health work in the United States, although reasons for delay vary. The common factor is the time required to mobilize initial support or inability to maintain support once a program is in operation.

The decades of delay in establishing a national animal health agency and in attacking CBPP have been discussed. National action to eliminate hog cholera was delayed even longer than for CBPP.

In the early 1900s BAI scientists identified the hog cholera virus and developed a hyperimmune anti-serum that could provide long-term immunity when administered simultaneously with virulent virus. The procedure was risky, as use of the virulent virus could spread the disease, but hog cholera was so damaging to the U.S. swine industry that the serum-virus procedure rapidly became the accepted method for trying to live with the disease. Under these conditions an eradication program was not feasible, and it was not until safer vaccines became available in the 1950s that public interest in eradication of the disease rose to a level that resulted in initiation of a program. In contrast the Canadians, who had not experienced the devastating outbreaks that had swept the United States, decided by 1900 to initiate an eradication program. One feature of the program was a decision that the risk from serum-virus use was too great to permit the procedure to be used in Canada.

The early history of bovine tuberculosis program work also demonstrates the time needed to arrive at a decision to act against a long-established disease. The first experimental use of tuberculin was in a dairy herd in 1891, the same year the BAI started large-scale production of tuberculin for use in testing. The *American Veterinary Review* reported widespread attention to tuberculosis and tuberculin. Sixteen years later (1907) the BAI chief told the American Veterinary Medical Association that it was time to face eradication of bovine tuberculosis, but that considerable work remained in order to gain support of cattle owners and the public; he was aware of the difference between having sufficient technical information and being able to put it to use on a large scale.

In 1911 a prevalence survey showed that the incidence of the disease had increased to as high as 14%. In 1917 a federal-state eradication program was started on an area-by-area basis. Appropriations were insufficient, resulting in the federal indemnity funds being exhausted in 1921. The program finally received new stimulus in 1925 when Chicago won a court case involving a city regulation requiring that milk coming into Chicago be from tested herds.

The campaign to eradicate bovine brucellosis, the costliest animal health program to date in U.S. history, reduced the national prevalence from an estimated 5% in 1947 (Manthei et al. 1956) to 0.9% of the 19.2 million cattle blood-tested in 1982 (Johnson 1982). The national effort against this disease started as an adjunct of a government-sponsored cattle reduction program in the drought and depression years (1930s); as long as cattle were going to be removed from production it would be sound practice to include brucellosis reactor animals. Not until after World War II, when estimated brucellosis infection doubled (Manthei et al. 1956), did the United States Animal Health Association and other interested groups muster sufficient political interest to enable legislative and financial support for the large-scale eradication effort that started in 1954.

Psoroptic scabies of sheep was so prevalent in the United States by the late 1800s that in 1896 Great Britain and other countries prohibited entry of U.S. sheep. In 1897 the disease was subjected to increasingly stringent regulatory measures. By 1942 only small areas in two states, where small flocks and frequent movements of small lots through markets made eradication difficult, remained under quarantine (Miller 1942).

Public indifference allowed the disease to remain a threat until 1960, when a concerted eradication effort was mounted that led to the last case being found in 1970: declaration of eradication was in 1973.

The elimination of scabies of cattle has a similarly long but less satisfactory history. Common throughout the range states by the early 1900s, the disease was addressed by the BAI and the states in 1904. Through a program of supervised dipping and quarantine, the disease was "practically eradicated," and by 1942 no areas remained under federal quarantine (Snyder 1942). Complacency over apparent success led to decreased inspections and reduced support for the regulatory measures required; the disease began to spread. Forty years later (1982) 115 outbreaks of psoroptic scabies of cattle were reported in 11 western and midwestern states, and through October 1982, scabies had been reported for 76 consecutive months (USAHA 1982).

Effective techniques for eliminating scabies have been known and demonstrated since the early 1900s. Nonetheless, sheep scabies persisted until the affected industry finally decided to allow the techniques to be properly applied. To date the cattle industry still is not sufficiently interested in eradicating the disease to support regulatory measures necessary to stamp it out.

It is not inevitable, however, that action against a dangerous and long established disease will be delayed long past the acquisition of the technical knowledge needed to act, or that support for the program will be insufficient. The eradication of cattle tick fever provides an example.

The "wasting fever" of eastern cattle in the late eighteenth and early nineteenth centuries and the "Texas fever" of western cattle drives in the Civil War era were the same disease and had long been observed to result from the introduction of apparently healthy southern cattle. In the West, fear of the disease led to private vigilante action, sometimes called shotgun quarantines, by northern stockmen. Although individual states adopted various regulatory restrictions, the infected zones kept moving farther north.

In 1889 the Secretary of Agriculture, in the first national quarantine order, established a federal quarantine line that allowed entry of southern cattle only for immediate slaughter. This checked northern spread of the disease but left the infected areas without help (McKeller 1942).

That same year BAI scientists demonstrated that the direct cause of the disease was a protozoan carried in the red blood cells of infected cattle. There had long been speculation by some western cattlemen that the cattle tick common to the southern states was involved in the cycle of the disease—an idea ridiculed by some of their peers. The BAI assigned Theobald Smith and F. L. Kilborne, who had identified the protozoan causing the disease, to study the tick. By 1890 they had demonstrated that southern cattle without ticks could not infect a pasture and that ticks alone, scattered on a pasture, could produce the disease. They also proved that blood from infected cattle would produce the disease when injected into susceptible animals. A third BAI veterinarian, Cooper Curtice, worked out the life cycle of the tick.

This led to speculation that cattle tick fever would disappear if the transmission cycle was broken by eliminating the tick. In 1897 a Texas rancher started dipping trials, in which the BAI participated, to find an effective tickicide. The next year federal quarantine procedures were altered to permit cattle, properly dipped in a sulfur and oil mixture, to move from a quarantined area without restriction. By 1906 feasibility studies of tick eradication led to inauguration of a nationwide program, which included 965 counties in 15 southern and southwestern states (McKeller 1942).

After a long and difficult program, the tick was eradicated in 1943. Although some areas along the Mexican border are still liable to encroachment by the tick, and a variety of the tick that can live on both deer and cattle has required periodic attention, cattle tick fever is no longer known in U.S. cattle.

With this disease, public concern was, and remained, strong enough to permit prompt implementation of new scientific information and to sustain the effort during a lengthy and sometimes violent campaign.

## Canada

The Dominion of Canada was established in 1869 when the British North America Act provided for confederation of the provinces. In 1869 the Contagious Diseases of Animals Act created a national veterinary authority, whose mission was to provide inspection of livestock at ports and along the Canadian–U.S. border. By the 1880s the annual report of the Chief Veterinary Inspector included both a review of import and export activities and a discussion of other significant events affecting animal health.

In 1881 the report noted that Canada remained free from all diseases of a contagious nature included in the Contagious Diseases of Animals Act—free to export to any port and market (Canada Dept. of Agriculture 1881). This was a definite marketing advantage, particularly since CBPP was still active in Europe and the United States.

That same year saw a controversy over FMD when U.S. slaughter cattle developed FMD en route to England in Canadian vessels. An investigation implicated the tie ropes used to restrain cattle on livestock ships. These ropes accompanied the cattle to the slaughterhouse in England, were replaced by ropes taken from cattle slaughtered earlier, and returned as part of the ships' equipment to North America for the next load. The assumption was that the ropes returned to the ships from the slaughterhouse were contaminated with FMD virus.

As a result, Canada adopted an Order in Council prohibiting the loading of any vessel in Canada that had carried cattle from U.S. ports until the ship had been cleaned, disinfected, and held for 30 or more days, depending on the disease history of animals previously shipped on that vessel.

While FMD had occasioned this action, the greatest apprehension in Canada was the risk of introducing CBPP. No U.S. cattle were permitted entry into Canada, although cattle from Great Britain, where CBPP was also endemic, could enter Canada subject to a 90-day quarantine.

The 1881 report also noted that anthrax was present in many parts of the dominion and the fear of introducing hog cholera from the United States required restricting U.S. swine to those for immediate slaughter under control.

**SHEEP SCABIES.** The British also reported in 1881 that scabies had been found in Canadian sheep that landed in Liverpool. The Chief Veterinary Inspector responded that no scabies could be found in Canada; however, the next year sheep scabies was found near Montreal. An 1882 Order in Council established a quarantine and dipping program, with a recommendation that all sheep for export from Canada receive a precautionary dipping (Canada Dept. of Agriculture 1882).

The establishment of regulatory requirements did not automatically solve the problem. In 1884 scabies was still present and the need to enforce the 1882 order was emphasized. In 1885 inspection and dipping activities were reported in four Quebec counties, and in 1886 there was a note that owners were "picking" their flocks to conceal the disease (Canada Dept. of Agriculture 1884, 1885, 1886).

Sheep scabies was finally eradicated from Canada in 1927 (Canada Dept. of Agriculture 1967), 45 years after the initial Order in Council but 46 years before eradication was achieved in the United States.

**FOOT-AND-MOUTH DISEASE.** Canadian experience with FMD in the 1800s was similar to that in the United States. The initial outbreak for both countries started in Canada in 1870 from cattle landed at Montreal (Canada Dept. of Agriculture 1903). The disease moved into New England but died out in both countries during that winter. In 1875 a disease diagnosed as FMD broke out near Toronto in imported sheep. There was some spread from this outbreak, but winter came to the rescue and the disease died out. There was an outbreak in 1884 in an import quarantine station with no spread.

No FMD was reported in Canada for over 60 years, until the disease appeared in Saskatchewan in 1952. The subsequent stamping-out program was concluded by mid-August, after slaughtering the animals on 29 infected and 13 contact premises. No specific source for this outbreak was established (Canada Dept. of Agriculture 1967).

**HOG CHOLERA.** Hog cholera was first recognized in Canada in the late summer of 1885 in southwest Quebec. At that time U.S. slaughter hogs were allowed entry into Canada, and the outbreak apparently resulted from a mix-up in Montreal when Canadian swine in transit were put in pens used for U.S. slaughter hogs. From Quebec the disease spread to Ontario, eventually involving 143 farms (Canada Dept. of Agriculture 1896).

By 1896 the disease spread to Toronto and Montreal, and an intensified slaughter program was adopted. However, the disease persisted in Ontario through 1903, and "stand-still" orders were issued in infected areas. In 1904, with 344 quarantines in Ontario, it was evident that the program was not effective in that province. After examination of what might be contributing to the persistence of the disease in southern Ontario, it was decided that procedures for moving U.S. swine from Michigan to New York across southern Ontario were too lax, including risks from manure scattered along the track system and the practice of hosing down in-transit hogs during the summer. Also noted was an incident in western Canada that year in which U.S. hogs in transit from North Dakota to Seattle left hog cholera behind in the Calgary yards when they were unloaded after a rail breakdown. In 1905 more stringent inspection and disinfection rules for rail cars were adopted, and later extended to trucks (Canada Dept. of Agriculture 1903, 1904, 1905).

Animal health officers recognized early the danger of feeding uncooked swill to swine and in 1898 recommended that all swill going to swine be boiled. Eighteen years later (1916) a regulation was introduced that required the cooking of swill fed to swine (McClanaghan 1961), 36 years before similar requirements began to be adopted in the United States. In 1913 Canada also decided not to permit hog cholera vaccination.

By these measures, and with a generation (1885–1905) required to stamp out persistent infection in parts of Ontario and Quebec, Canada has remained free from endemic hog cholera without vaccination and at a low relative cost compared to the expense of continued vaccination and endemic disease. This was done in spite of allowing imports of U.S. pork to meet consumption demands. A large outbreak in southern Quebec in 1960–1961, just prior to initiation of the U.S. hog cholera eradication program, required a stand-still order and stamping-out program over a large area.

**CONTAGIOUS BOVINE PLEUROPNEUMONIA.** In the nineteenth century, though CBPP was of great concern in Europe and the United States, it was never introduced into Canada. However, the risk of an introduction was a constant worry to Canadian animal health officials until the disease was eliminated from western Europe and the United States at the end of the 1800s. From 1843 to 1892 the danger of infection across the U.S.–Canadian border was constant, and during those same years the growing Canadian cattle industry required European bloodlines, which necessitated not only the importing of animals but also a quarantine policy that prevented introduction of the disease.

In 1886 CBPP appeared in cattle en route to Canada from Scotland. Two hundred head were destroyed in the Canadian import quarantine station; 37 cattle adjacent to the station were killed as a precautionary measure. There was no extension of the disease either within or without the station (Canada Dept. of Agriculture 1886). In 1892 the British, who at that time were trying to complete their CBPP eradication program, reported CBPP in a shipment of Canadian stocker cattle and embargoed further shipments except animals for immediate slaughter. In spite of Canadian protest that there had never been evidence of CBPP in Canada, the embargo lasted until 1923 (Canada Dept. of Agriculture 1967).

Canada and the United States, with a 4000-mile open border and similar livestock industries on both sides of that border, have followed similar patterns in attacking many animal diseases common to both countries. In 1897 a formal Canadian–U.S. agreement was made for immediate notification of outbreaks of contagious diseases, which resulted in withdrawal of the 90-day-entry quarantine each country had previously required. Tuberculin was first used in Canada in 1894 on an experimental farm, an accredited-herd plan was introduced in 1919, and area tuberculosis testing started in 1923. Bovine brucellosis control started in 1957, shortly after the accelerated eradication program was initiated in the United States (Canada Dept. of Agriculture 1967).

The Canadian Health of Animals organization has, since its inception in 1869, remained a respected support for Canadian agriculture. In 1967 a commemorative publication stated that "among the many services offered by the Department of Agriculture, none has a longer or more distinguished history than the work done under the Contagious Diseases of Animals Act" (Canada Dept. of Agriculture 1967).

## Latin America and the Caribbean

From northern Mexico and the Bahamas to the Antarctic approaches, the Latin American and Caribbean communities cover a distance equivalent to that from San Francisco to Tokyo or New York to Athens.

The 35 countries and dependencies in this area had their modern political origins in European colonial expansion from the sixteenth through the eighteenth centuries, with Spain leaving behind the overwhelming cultural influence. Although Spain looked on these colonies as a source of treasure, the other colonizers, especially in the Caribbean, developed these tropical areas as producers of plantation crops for export. Large-scale livestock production came later, primarily in Latin America, where meat and animal products have become significant export items for many countries.

Of the approximately 500 million hectares of agricultural land in the region, 400 million (80%) are suitable for pasturage and animal production. The United States, with about the same number of hectares for agricultural production, uses only 55% as pasturage.

The importance of livestock to Latin America is shown by the establishment of faculties of veterinary medicine in several universities by the early twentieth century. Cultural and language ties resulted in these schools aligning themselves with their predecessors in Spain and Italy. As with veterinary schools elsewhere, the emphasis was on curing disease and was directed toward individuals or individual herds.

During the twentieth century there has been growing interest in regional exchanges on preventive medicine and large-scale disease control. The first multinational conference on FMD in the Western Hemisphere was called by Panama in 1951, after the FMD virus invaded the Andean countries and threatened countries to the north.

In 1951 the Pan-American Health Organization, upon request from the Organization of American States, established in collaboration with the Inter-American Institute on Agricultural Sciences, the Center for FMD in Rio de Janiero. In 1956 the Center for Zoonoses was created in Buenos Aires. Early efforts were restricted to applied research, technical assistance, and training. One of the most noteworthy research results, in collaboration with Plum Island Animal Disease Center, came with the development of an improved vaccine for FMD. Training in FMD-related subjects has included professional graduates from 36 countries.

Within Latin America, FMD provides the most significant and dramatic difference between the "have" and "have-not" nations. Latin American countries from Panama north through Mexico have been able to remain free of endemic FMD. For practical purposes, Chile is the only South American country to carry out a national eradication program.

Chile, in recent years, carried out a successful national FMD eradication program. To date their FMD-free status has been challenged once by an introduction of the disease in the high mountain summer pasture area along the Andean border with Argentina. The Chilean animal health agency maintains an organized program in these areas to detect and eliminate such introductions. The northeastern countries of Surinam, Guyana, and French Guiana are normally FMD free but on occasion may be subjected to introductions across their river and forestland borders. For control, Latin American countries with endemic FMD depend heavily on virus-typing support from the Rio center and vaccine programs.

The largest effort to eradicate FMD north of the Panamanian-Columbian border took place in Mexico from 1946 to 1954 (16 states in central Mexico). Over the years the program, conducted in cooperation with the United States, combined slaughter, vaccination, and quarantine before finally succeeding. Over 1 million animals were slaughtered and about 60 million doses of vaccine were used for systematic vaccination. At the height of the program, 6000 Mexican and 2000 U.S. BAI personnel plus 5000 Mexican soldiers were utilized.

That this monumental effort persisted until successfully concluded is an illustration of the dedication of all the countries north of South America to the principle that FMD will not be allowed to become established. The fact that the Panamanian-Columbian border is the dividing line between free and infected areas results in some differences of opinion in handling the problem. In recent years these differences have crystallized the concern in Panama and north over completion of the last link of the Pan-American highway, which if constructed, would for the first time open up a natural barrier of jungle and swamp. The difference in interpretation of goals, whether the disease is to be controlled or eradicated, is reviewed in more depth in Chapter 2.

To date the only known introduction of African swine fever into a continental country in the Americas occurred in Brazil in the late 1970s — a matter of concern to all the countries in the region. No additional cases were reported from Brazil in the most recent reporting year (1984).

The tropical and subtropical climates of many Latin American countries lead to the persistence of animal diseases that thrive in such surroundings. Ticks and tick-borne diseases such as bovine piroplasmosis result in large economic losses. Transmission of rabies through vampire bat species, consumers of blood meals, is not only of concern to humans but also, as in other tropical areas, is a constant threat to livestock, particularly those that range freely at night.

The larvae of the warble fly (*Hypoderma lineatum*) are damaging parasites of cattle in the United States and Canada. From central Mexico through South America ranges another species (*Dermatobia hominis*), called "torsalo," "moyacuil," and other local names, whose larval form causes lesions in livestock similar to the "ox warbles" found farther north.

In recent years Mexico and the United States have been involved in a campaign to eradicate the "screwworm" fly (*Cochliomyia hominovorax*). Until recently this pest, whose eggs are laid in wounds and produce larvae that consume living tissue, had a year-round range from frost-free areas in south Texas and Florida to deep into South America. During the summer months the flies spread farther as the temperatures rose. Since the fly mates only once, the introduction by airdrop of artificially reared and sterilized flies, along with other supporting techniques, succeeded in eliminating overwintering populations in the United States by the early 1970s. Now a cooperative program in Mexico, with a fly-rearing facility at the narrow Isthmus of Tehuantepec in southern Mexico, is designed to eradicate the fly from all of Mexico north of the Isthmus.

The Caribbean countries and dependencies are low in land mass and relatively high in population; consequently the area is heavily dependent on imported food, particularly protein sources. As livestock populations are low in relation to the number of people, productivity is therefore important. Significant livestock disease is particularly damaging in such an environment, and preventing the establishment of exotic disease is of prime concern to animal health agencies. FMD has been kept out, and the story of African swine fever (ASF) in the Caribbean is an example of this concern.

ASF was diagnosed in Cuba in 1971. Cuban veterinary authorities moved swiftly into an area-quarantine and stamping-out program, which was successful; 33 centers of infection were found and over 20,000 swine slaughtered. A subsequent ASF outbreak in Cuba was also eliminated, but later in the decade ASF was found in the Dominican Republic and then in Haiti, the two countries that share the island of Hispaniola east of Cuba.

With assistance from other countries in the Western Hemisphere, the two countries attacked the problem through total depopulation of swine, followed by a "vacation" period and then gradual and controlled repopulation. This Draconean procedure had the added potential advantage of making it possible to rebuild a swine population free of hog cholera as well as ASF.

The Caribbean countries and dependencies, as could be expected, face the usual disease problems found in livestock populations of European origin (i.e., bovine brucellosis and tuberculosis). In addition, they face the types of disease and parasite problems found in tropical areas. Since there is an ever increasing flow of people and products to these islands due to their popularity with vacationers, the risk from introduced disease remains high.

The Latin American and Caribbean countries, many with past and continuing economic difficulties and political unrest and located in hot climates that provide no vacation from disease, to date have been able to prevent the establishment of many of the animal disease plagues existing in other parts of the world. An important factor in animal health activities has been the work of multinational organizations such as the Pan-American Health Organization, the Inter-American Institute for Cooperation in Agriculture, and the Interregional Organization for Livestock and Agricultural Health which have provided not only the initiative for continuing multinational discussion but also field and laboratory support. Strong financial support for the animal health programs has come from such organizations as the International Development Bank.

# 6

# Program-timing Factors

THERE ARE TWO CLASSES of disease control or eradication programs. One is an emergency effort against a newly introduced agent or the sudden explosion of one already present — essentially defensive reactions after the fact. The other is an offensive, preplanned, nonemergency program against an established pathogen. These latter programs are planned in advance and initiated at a time and level primarily determined by those agencies responsible for the campaign.

The differing circumstances between these two classes result in differences in timing. If an emergency program is to be successful, the speed of reaction to the emergency is vital. Preplanned, nonemergency programs usually develop slowly, after long periods of deliberation, and often long after the accumulation of sufficient scientific and technical knowledge provides reasonable assurance of success.

Experienced health administrators know that the same public that will accept, even demand, immediate action against a new and explosive disease will resist initiating a program against a long-established disease. Individuals and groups (including governments) are resistant to change and proper program timing requires recognition of this fact.

Public demand for speedy action in a health emergency results from an unwillingness to accept a new threat to accustomed patterns. When dealing with an established disease in livestock and poultry operations, the adjustments necessitated by disease have long been accomplished. Producers may grumble over the continuing losses but accept the problem since production and marketing has adjusted to allow coexistence. When a disease control or eradication program is eventually advocated, there is an initial reluctance to change the accustomed way of doing things, particularly when future quarantines, added restrictions on shipping animals and commercial products, and the other less-than-pleasant aspects of a regulatory program are being considered. Enthusiasm rarely accompanies uncertainty.

Any health professional who has been involved in trying to launch a program against an established disease of major significance has been frustrated at times by the disinterest, apathy, or even opposition of many individuals or groups who would benefit from such a program. It is important to remember that a long period of discussion and evolution of attitudes is required to overcome resistance to change.

Health professionals need to understand and be a part of this evolution of attitude. They need this time to learn the interests, requirements, and capabilities of the many groups that will be involved in a large program so they can expand their own understanding beyond their fields of technical specialization.

Because of the variety and complexity of the nonmedical aspects of program planning, initiation, and operation, it is sometimes tempting for health protection professionals to be concerned only with their own specialized input to a program, leaving the rest to someone else. This is a mistake. Experienced health professionals are the persons best equipped to weigh scientific requirements against the needs and capacities of other interests and to judge the overall probability of success for the proposed program. A balanced judgment requires not only a knowledge of disease but also an understanding of the political, economic, and social relationships of those involved.

## Foundations of Support

In an emergency health program there is little time available to build a foundation of public interest. The only real questions in program timing are (1) whether or not sufficient technical capability exists with which to start a program and (2) if there is adequate public (political) demand for action present. If public demand is not quickly evident, it is probable that the initial emergency will become an established disaster. Therefore, health program administrators need to judge technical capabilities quickly and, if the answer is positive, recommend immediate and massive responses.

For reasons already discussed, the time for foundation building is expanded when considering a planned program against an established pathogen. Legislators and heads of government must be convinced that persistent disease is, in fact, too expensive or too much of a risk to public health to go unchallenged, e.g., the smallpox eradication program. Although no case had been reported in the United States since 1949 (Cent. Disease Control 1979a), the annual cost of prevention to the nation was estimated at $140 million in 1969 (Axnick and Lane 1972). However, when the decision was made to support a worldwide eradication program, the cost was only $27 million (Cent. Disease Control 1979b).

Public demand alone for a campaign against an established disease agent will not be sufficient; those affected by the disease must be aroused to the point that they influence the policymakers. Governments act when an alliance of interest groups makes a case for the proposed program strong enough so that it cannot be ignored — a case that is stronger than any presented by other interests seeking political and/or economic support for competing endeavors. A single government agency, such as a health protection organization, can seldom expect to exert sufficient influence to bring about a new program when acting alone.

Compared with human populations, domestic livestock and poultry are captive populations that can be controlled and manipulated. As a result, there is more historical information on control and eradication programs for animal diseases than for human diseases. The factors involved in preprogram consensus building can be drawn from these histories.

For animal health programs, the alliance of interest groups that is needed includes the affected segments of the livestock or poultry industry in addition to veterinary organizations, academia, meat or poultry processors, transportation and marketing interests, and government agencies. Each group will be involved for different reasons; some will offer support, some will speak in opposition, and others will support only a particular portion of the program. Each is likely to favor restrictions on someone else but not on their own group.

Therefore, a consensus must develop on what must be done, both technically in structuring an operational plan and politically in getting the plan authorized, funded, and initiated, regardless of whether funds come from the national government or from a mix of government, industry, and international financing. Development of this consensus is critical to final success. If the many interests involved cannot agree on an overall program that is technically sound, any program that is initiated will encounter difficulty. And when dealing with disease programs, the health protection agencies must be included and must take an active part, if for no other reason than to avoid implementing a technically unsound program or one that calls for actions beyond the capacity of those who must carry it out.

A satisfactory foundation for a health program exists when there is (1) a pronounced economic or public health impact, (2) a sustained interest on the part of affected public groups, (3) a willingness to accept change, (4) sufficient scientific knowledge to give reasonable hope of success, (5) cooperation among governmental bodies, and (6) adequate financial resources.

**IMPACT OF DISEASE.** Food-animal medicine is based squarely on economics, whether for large public programs or for determining treatment protocols for an individual animal or herd. Livestock owners are not greatly concerned over a disease that does not exert damaging economic effects on their operations. In 1947 prior to the initiation of an accelerated effort to eradicate *Brucella abortus* from the United States, reported cases of brucellosis in humans reached 6321 (National Brucellosis Technical Commission 1978b). However, to gain support from cattle owners for the coming campaign, the U.S. Livestock Sanitary Association stressed the estimated $100 million annual loss that the cattlemen were already suffering from the disease.

Historically, public perception of the degree of economic loss caused by a disease has been based on impressions from direct observation by livestock owners. Also, structured analyses of economic losses that are now expected in developing cost/benefit studies for government use are valuable for convincing industry that a disease is, in fact, causing significant economic damage. As the use of such studies has grown for proposed government programs, including health programs, the economic analysis required is much more sophisticated than was necessary in earlier years.

Health professionals usually are not economists and do not have the training to construct economic models. On the other hand, economists are not health professionals and do not have knowledge of disease and the sociopolitical constraints surrounding the initiation and conduct of health protection programs. Proper analysis of data requires both types of knowledge. Health professionals, therefore need to be familiar with the economic modeling process in order to function effectively as a member of the multidisciplinary team that is required to complete the type of comprehensive study needed prior to instituting a large program.

These studies are now required prior to approval and funding of most public programs. The time required to develop the model must be taken into account in considering the time frame for a new program, not only in the timing of a program against an established disease, but also in planning for future emergency situations. A preliminary economic analysis of the potential impact of a dangerous exotic disease can save vital time if the emergency actually develops.

Production cycles can also be an important consideration in the timing of control or eradication efforts. For example, when economic or climatic conditions are reducing herd sizes, a prime opportunity exists for selective culling. This situation led to initiation of a brucellosis control program in the United States in 1934, during a period of lengthy drought and economic depression. Condemnation and depopulation are far more acceptable in times such as these, especially if indemnity funds are available. In addition, a far greater percentage of herd culls go to slaughter rather than to other herds, thus reducing the amount of interherd exposure.

Conversely, when producers increase their herd size, they are eager to acquire more breeding stock and resist condemnation efforts. Building herd size also results in fewer closed herds, increased interherd transfers of livestock, less discriminating purchases, greater reluctance to comply with restrictive regulatory requirements, and wider dissemination of pathogens.

For a practitioner of human medicine, life and health maintenance are beyond economic value judgements when determining the cost effectiveness of treatment. This reflects the view of the clientele — that human life, particularly our own, is priceless. For a practitioner of food-animal medicine the prime concern is economic. His clients are livestock owners who maintain their animals for economic rather than emotional reasons. Disease, however, cannot be divided neatly to conform to these biases. Communicable diseases of concern to humans cannot be considered in exclusively human terms; there are over 150 zoonoses, diseases transmitted naturally between other animals and humans (Hubbert et al. 1975).

The medical professions, however, do not yet fully realize that human and nonhuman health problems are so closely intertwined. This may be due in part to differing concerns regarding the impact of disease, with one group looking at human health and the other at economic loss. Consumers of animal products feel that they deserve protection from disease risk when using these products. However, producers are inclined to think first in terms of making a profit from their operation. Human health risk may be of little real concern to producers unless the regulatory steps taken to protect public health interfere with their economic return.

These differing areas of primary interest need to be recognized and taken into consideration in planning disease control or eradication programs. When discussing the potential value of a program, consumer groups are interested in the public health aspects and possibly the potential benefits to wildlife. The producers of food animals will be far more interested in the expected economic impact of the program.

**PUBLIC DEMAND.** Proper program timing requires adequate technical knowledge plus sufficient public demand and support. Acquisition of knowledge does not automatically ensure demand, and public concern over the ravages of a disease does not necessarily translate into support for an effective control or eradication program. Those involved in health protection must not cause undue public concern, but must obtain understanding of, and support for, the requirements of large-scale health programs.

An initial step for a program planner is to define the groups or individuals that are most affected by the disease, as well as those that will be affected by a control or eradication program. Obviously, these groups will vary with different diseases, depending on the species specificity of the agent and whether or not there is human health risk. Identification of these groups is important, though it may seem elementary. In developmental stages of a program, it is a dilution of effort to try to involve segments of the general public that will have only a peripheral interest in the disease or in the impact of the program.

Once this "interested public" has been determined, it is necessary to evaluate the level of demand for a control or eradication program — remembering again that fear of a disease does not necessarily translate into high-level support. Witness the worldwide concern over foot-and-mouth disease and the relatively few countries that, up to now, have been seriously interested in undertaking the rigors required in an eradication program.

If demand for a program is limited, the program should not be initiated until there has been a strong effort to present the problem and the proposed plans for action. To achieve success it is important that affected groups unite to support the goal of the program, otherwise there is no real base for progress.

This is illustrated by experience in the United States with equine infectious anemia (EIA). There is no public health threat from EIA, thus it would seem to present the ideal set of circumstances around which to develop an eradication program. EIA affects only one species; is usually manifested as an acute disease with a high case-fatality rate; presently has a low incidence in most parts of the country; is detectable by a rapid, accurate, and economical diagnostic test; and is recognized by the equine industry as a major disease threat.

Even though the adverse impact of the disease is recognized and there is ample technical knowledge to enable eradication of EIA, to date the various elements of the equine industry have not shown a coordinated and aggressive support for a large-scale regulatory program. Since EIA has no public health significance, without united support from the industry there has been no reason for government agencies to initiate action to eradicate the virus.

In contrast, hog cholera virus, which also affects only one domestic species and has no public health significance, has been eradicated from the United States. The most important factor in the success of that program was the dedication of the leaders of the swine industry to eradication—a dedication that was maintained before and throughout the program despite strong initial opposition from some swine producers, veterinarians, and government officials.

If the target pathogen presents a public health risk, the definition of "interested public" is enlarged to include those people at greatest risk. Inclusion of the general public is seldom indicated or productive at this stage of program development. For example, it would be practical and justifiable to discuss with slaughterhouse workers, stock handlers, and veterinarians the specific risk to them from brucellosis-infected cattle. It would not be justifiable to start a publicity campaign directed toward the general public implying a significant risk to all from this bacterium.

In an effort to eliminate *Cysticercus bovis* from a cattle population, it would be foolhardy and unnecessary to try to arouse support for a program to screen the entire human population for *Taenia saginata* just because humans are the only host of the adult form of this cattle parasite. The human targets for involvement in the proposal can be limited to those who handle cattle, as bovine infection comes from inadequate personal sanitation practices by infected cattle handlers.

**SCIENTIFIC AND TECHNICAL INFORMATION.** Scientific and technical adequacy must be determined prior to the start of a health protection program, and although advice from many sources is required, the responsibility properly rests with the agency that will be conducting the program.

Advice from two extremes can be expected. Those who strongly desire a program will recommend moving quickly with the expectation of solving technical questions as they arise. Those in opposition will often advise that, while they do not oppose the general idea of a program, there should be no action until additional research has been conducted. This argument always appears in presentations against a new program. It should be remembered that there is never a full range of knowledge about any pathogen, including those that have already been eradicated from one or more countries. Both of these extreme positions may sound convincing to those who are inexperienced in health programs, however, each avoids the real task of defining the minimum level of knowledge needed to initiate the type of program contemplated and determining if that level has been reached. That task is best carried out by health protection professionals.

The abilities to find and confine or eliminate foci of infection are technical factors to be considered in arriving at a decision. Some of the questions that need to be addressed are

1. Is there a diagnostic procedure sufficiently specific and sensitive (yet practical) for program use, including speed of obtaining results and the ability to detect carriers?

2. How much confidence can be placed in the accuracy and adequacy of reports of disease occurrence?

3. Are there epidemiologic studies applicable to the area where the program will be conducted, including the ability of wild species to act as reservoirs or transmitters or the agent?

4. Are the most frequent routes of transmission known?

5. Can the causative agent be destroyed on site or from contaminated materials by known disinfection procedures?

Another factor to be considered is the effect of vaccination on the type of program contemplated. Here, the following questions must be addressed.

1. Are presently available vaccines sufficiently efficacious in preventing infection rather than just masking clinical evidence of disease?

2. What is the risk of agent spread by vaccines now in use?

3. Can the vaccines significantly confuse interpretation of diagnostic tests?

These factors cannot properly be considered individually. Technical sufficiency of the total must be based on many units of information. Prudence is necessary to prevent unwarranted optimism, but an overly cautious approach may prevent action on a worthwhile program.

Although the agency operating the program should decide the level of scientific information required to initiate a program, that agency needs to work with the scientific community to evaluate the question. Preferably, interaction should be on a direct basis and not confined solely to a study of published research material for the following reasons:

1. Mutual understanding of the problems and needs for the program must be developed.

2. Exposure to information not contained in published reports, particularly negative research results, can provide important background information for program planners.

3. Stimulation of scientific study of the problem may lead to possible support for research study with resources available to the program agency.

4. Interaction may stimulate support for the program objectives from scientists experienced in the field.

Ideally, the time to seek research experience bearing on a program is while the program is being developed rather than waiting until it is in operation, particularly if the acquired information raises questions about the scientific validity of planned operational procedures.

An agency whose mission is the planning and operation of health protection programs seldom has the competence, funds, personnel, or authority to engage in basic research. When a new program is being considered within the agency, comprehensive knowledge of research bearing on the disease is usually incomplete. While a literature search for relevant material is necessary and useful, this material will not necessarily be directly related to program questions.

Direct communication with researchers will expand the scientific background of program planners and may lead to further contacts. Since disease control and eradication programs involve problems too complex to handle by individual effort and cover wide geographic areas, the scientific questions facing program planners are never simple.

Politically, a program agency must put its proposals in competition with other agencies that are requesting funds for other purposes. Health protection programs are regulatory, hence restrictive in nature; thus political opposition is aroused by those who anticipate interference with their usual method of operation. A ploy often used by opponents of a proposed program is to criticize the proposal as scientifically unsound. A defense offered solely by the program agency may be regarded as biased. If the proposed program plans have been reviewed and favorably judged by qualified scientists, the program agency will have objective scientific support for the proposal.

A good example of this early and continued cooperation between program directors and research scientists is the U.S.-Mexican screwworm eradication program, which was started in 1962 in the southwestern United States and northern Mexico and later moved to southern Mexico. Throughout this massive effort the joint policy planning between field program directors and research scientists has continued; the research units continue to assist in improving operational procedures.

## Elements of Decision Making

Since health protection programs are large-scale efforts, it is essential that program directors comprehend the complexities that comprise the total program.

No program director or agency head can expect to be expert in all fields. They must be able to judge whether or not the assembled information provides a sound basis for proceeding, and they need a system that will assist them in discerning significant deficiencies or misinformation in the important interest areas.

Scientific fields of inquiry are becoming ever more specialized — socioeconomic factors are increasing in number and complexity as cultures change and expand. Yet the decision maker, who usually functions as a generalist, must gather this diverse information into a cohesive whole to make a judgment on the potential success and timing of the total effort. The scope of the assembled information can be bewildering if viewed as an uncatalogued collection of facts. Sound overall evaluation may be made even more difficult by the intentional or unintentional desire of individual staff advisors or consultants to present their area of special interest as the most important part of the total.

Therefore, the approach to final decision making is not to attempt expertise in all fields but to develop a systematic organization and evaluation of the assembled information. As a result of specialized studies in the field of administration, there are a variety of systems available aimed at structured decision making. All these systems are designed to provide an orderly procedure for choosing alternatives, which is the essence of decision making. The systems were developed to meet differing needs and are named accordingly.

*Planning-Programing-Budgeting Systems (PPBS)* — was designed to facilitate allocation of resources without regard to implementation or evaluation (Gorham 1967)

*Operations research* — is a method for choosing, by a modeling procedure, the optimum use of resources by reducing operational trial and error through advanced selection of the most efficient combination of activities (Flagle 1963).

*Linear programing* — uses mathematical models to evaluate the expected results from various alternatives. It can be used to assist in determining optimal strategies.

*Systems analysis* — first developed by Chestnut (1965), may play a role in any of the above but is a more complex technique than those previously mentioned. The procedure is aimed at sorting out the relative significance of the important factors connected with the program or problem under study. Computer analyses, including changes in assumptions involving one or more factors, makes this approach more practical for general use than when calculations were largely manual.

*Benefit/cost and cost/effectiveness analyses* — are used to evaluate the expected social value in relation to the expenditure of public funds. While essentially economic, a sound end result also requires inclusion of noneconomic data relevant to the program. Simulation modeling is a more complex technique (Naylor et al. 1966) in which the expansion or retraction of a disease in a population is modeled by computer techniques, enabling estimates of the effect of various alternative control strategies. It has the advantages of flexibility and of closely approximating biological situations (Morris and Roe 1975).

These procedures are only tools, not sacred formulas, to assist the decision makers confronted with a mass of information relevant to a large health protection program. The directors must systematically examine the broadest range of knowledge that will enable them to wisely use those tools, for no system is successful in the hands of the uninformed or in the absence of essential facts.

# 7

## Keeping Disease Out

U.S. SECRETARY OF STATE GEORGE MARSHALL said that the only way to win a war is to prevent it. Similarly, the optimal method for handling disease is to prevent it. Disease control and eradication programs, while often dramatic, in reality are the result of failed prevention programs.

While all countries recognize the need for general disease prevention for their citizens, livestock, and domestic crops, the degree to which these needs are met depends primarily on the economic well-being of the society. Less affluent nations are continually burdened with disease, which inhibits domestic progress and threatens other societies. Although multinational efforts against disease have increased in recent years, they usually are directed against specific problems; general disease prevention remains a national or local responsibility.

In terms of national disease prevention, keeping out pathogens means preventing their introduction from a foreign source. Only a country that can maintain complete isolation can be free of such risks. For a variety of political, economic, and geographic factors, no human society of any size has existed in this fashion for many centuries, and in recent generations the rate and volume of international exchange of people, animals, and products has increased. A few nations are located on islands or peninsulas, facilitating border protection, but most countries share long land borders with other nations, making total quarantines virtually impossible.

The economic necessity for international movement of livestock was summarized by Wells (1978), who stated that the future development of livestock production hinges on the availability of an international basis of genetic material of recognized performance, regardless of the country of origin. For other economic reasons, the same is true for trade in animal products between regions of surplus production and those that fall short of domestic needs.

Consequently, national import quarantine procedures have been developed to reduce risk of exposure to foreign disease agents while, at the same time, permitting the exchange of people and property. Since domestic animals and animal products are more easily subjected to international quarantine procedures than are people, it is usually more cumbersome to move livestock or animal products across borders than it is for people to cross those same borders.

## Basic Systems for Import Control

There are two basic systems used to control imports. One is interdiction, where everything is prohibited—any shipment that is permitted entry comes in only after compliance with specific requirements designed for that shipment alone. The other is a system in which general standards are established—any shipment that qualifies is permitted entry. In effect, many countries use a combination of the two, reserving interdiction for proposed shipments from high-risk areas and general standards for shipments from less dangerous sources.

It is evident that interdiction provides tighter control, whereas preset general standards facilitate planning for ongoing commercial trade. Both systems should take into account risk factors such as the characteristics of diseases of concern, disease status of the originating and receiving countries, and routes of shipment. The route of shipment is important because it relates to the prevention of en route exposure and reduces the potential for shipping from infected areas through neutral zones, which can create confusion over the true nation of origin.

Attempts at keeping a pathogen out of a country generally result in differences between advocates of minimum restraint in international trade and government agencies, which have disease prevention as their primary objective. When dealing with diseases of domestic animals, advocates of minimum restraint are usually commercial interests involved in international trade. Government import restrictions tend to be supported by domestic livestock and poultry interests, who fear introduction of foreign pathogens and, to some extent, foreign economic competition.

Gradations of risk range from limiting imports to those directly from countries free of the pathogen of concern to accepting imports from a country where the agent is endemic. National health protection agencies try to adhere to the safest source of imports, but they may be forced to accept alternative choices because of economic or political factors; official agencies must search for a system of prevention with minimal compromise with safety.

Health protection officials can expect accusations of obstructionism and bureaucratic interference for their conservative policies, but adherence to such attitudes is an important part of their responsibility. Unless the heads of government agencies resist pressures, commercial interests with short-term objectives may pressure them into actions that could lead to national health problems.

Dealing with conflicting demands can result in compromise and development of new regulations that allow importation by providing safety margins not previously thought possible, e.g., the history of the movement of breeding cattle into North America from countries with foot-and-mouth disease (FMD).

Historically, the three North American countries have maintained a general policy of prohibiting entry of livestock from infected countries. However, in 1930 the United States strengthened its exclusion policy by adopting prohibitory legislation banning entry of domestic ruminants and swine from any country determined to have FMD. Canada and Mexico had a similar policy but did not adopt specific national prohibitory legislation.

After World War II North American cattle producers needed to increase production to meet international competition, and they wanted a way to introduce new genetic material from countries with FMD. Canada, using a combination of maximum security pre- and postentry quarantine plus new research breakthroughs in diagnostic procedures, inaugurated such a system in 1965. In 1970 the United States started a semen importation system based on similar quarantine procedures and, in more recent years, amended the 1930 prohibitory legislation to permit entry of live animals under specified conditions. The flow of new germ plasm to North America, including Mexico, through Canada, and the United States, has provided a minimum-risk method for North American cattle producers to upgrade their breeding herds. It seems probable that the current situation would not have developed without economic pressures to alter a prohibitory policy and without insistence on cautious change based on assured safety by health protection agencies.

The development of embryo-transfer techniques has opened a multitude of new opportunities for transfer of desirable genetic material, but to date, there is virtually no hard data on the potential of this technique for excluding or transmitting pathogens (Stringfellow et al. 1982).

Accepting the necessity for international exchange, the recipient country is, in reality, engaged in reducing disease risk rather than in absolute prevention; thus, the capabilities of the country of origin become an essential part of the process.

Since keeping pathogens out of a country is a responsibility of the national government, the regulation of imports cannot be properly exercised by international, local, or private interests. Similarly, the health protection agency of a receiving country must depend on the appropriate national health agency of the exporting country in determining the credibility of documentation provided at the point of origin. If the credibility is in doubt, the receiving country would be foolish to proceed unless it can have its own observers at the originating point, which is not only cumbersome and expensive, but is not the best basis for mutual confidence. One of the strongest commercial assets an exporting country can have as far as animals and animal products are concerned is a national veterinary service that has established an excellent reputation for professional competence and integrity. For example, Canada has safely imported cattle from European countries that have FMD because of a thorough knowledge of the veterinary services and FMD programs of the exporting countries (Wells 1968).

The importing country should base its import health requirements on scientific evidence of need for the purpose intended. However, import requirements that go beyond the bounds of scientific need or justification have sometimes been established. Bartlett (1978) pointed out that this can extend beyond meaningless "red tape," such as recertification of signatures of the responsible government official at origin by several levels of judicial and diplomatic rubber stamping, which in itself may be a procedural cover-up for incapacity in the original technical determination. Testing requirements that are without real value in disease prevention may be imposed; for example, regulations requiring that imported semen must originate from bulls negative to a tuberculin test within 30 days of semen collection. Frequent application (more than once each 6 months) of intradermal tuberculosis testing may produce negative results (nonreactors) in tuberculous cattle, therefore, the supplier can ship only semen produced during a few months each year or can administer tuberculin tests every 30 days year round; the test results would be "bureaucratically satisfying but technically meaningless and potentially dangerous."

Keeping pathogens out of an importing country depends on cooperative actions by both the importing and exporting countries. National health agencies in each country, while necessarily and primarily concerned with their own interests, can often negotiate differences in regulatory requirements if each has knowledge of the capabilities of the other country.

## Technical Aspects of Import Control

Sharman (1978) listed 12 techniques that could be applied in keeping pathogens out of a country: permits; health certificates; inspection at port of entry; quarantine of suppliers, with prohibition of entry of infected and exposed animals; isolation at recipient farms; entry only of disease-free animals; entry only from disease-free countries; quarantine at port of embarkation; laboratory examination; sentinel animals; treatment for ectoparasites; and vaccination. Antimicrobial treatment, as practiced in psittacosis control (Arnstein et al. 1968), can be added to the list. The last three techniques are of value only against a few disease agents.

Requesting an import permit serves the primary purpose of alerting the receiving nation to the fact that importation is intended and provides lead time, if needed, to establish prerequisite conditions for entry. If permits are issued merely as clerical functions without additional requirements or without adequate border policing, they are of no value in disease control.

Health certificates, properly worded and issued, can assist in averting entry of sick and exposed animals but are of limited value if they are issued merely on the basis of freedom from obvious clinical disease without due regard for the true health status of the animal. Other potential weaknesses are that identification of disease may be haphazard, and earlier exposures to disease may be unknown to, or concealed by, the seller. Improper certification, especially if fraudulent, should result in confiscation of the shipment or return at the shipper's expense. Imported stock is only as good as its certification.

Animals destined for import must be clearly and uniquely identified in a way that cannot be counterfeited and must be the only animals aboard the vessel or aircraft. The transport and its fittings plus all bedding, feed, water, and pens for the animals during shipping should be from the importing country or be sterilized. Carriers should not stop in infected countries because of the danger of pathogens being introduced to the cargo via feed, water, bedding, or personnel. They also must not stop in the importing country before the animals are disembarked at the designated entry point. The carrier should be disinfected and disinsecticized before proceeding. Special precautions must be taken with garbage accumulated during the trip.

Animals imported from a country with significant endemic disease exotic to the importing country should be imported only if they have great genetic value. Though the diversity and value of the gene pool of certain wild species and domestic breeds that have developed over the centuries in small corners of the earth cannot be denigrated, their worth should be evaluated and clearly documented before risking their introduction. With breeding stock, restricting entry to virgin animals will eliminate venereal pathogens.

Animal products present special problems because many preservation techniques such as refrigeration, freezing, and curing tend to preserve the pathogens as well. Procedures that preserve taste and texture are unlikely to destroy pathogens. At this time only heat can be relied on to render the product safe. As a new processing or packaging technique is developed, it should be tested with a multitude of pathogens and products. Canned meat or products carried by individuals must be prohibited because of the ease of tampering. There are scores of examples where labels or even contents of cans have been substituted. Amnesty bins should be provided at all ports of entry so that debarking passengers can discard meat or meat products without fear of prosecution. The cargo compartments of all air and ocean carriers transporting meat from countries with pathogens such as FMD or rinderpest should be emptied and disinfected before reaching disease-free nations.

A change in a nation's livestock disease status can cause an immediate reallocation of international trade due to the relatively small volume involved (Doyle 1979). For example, international trade consumes only 6% of the world beef supply; therefore, there are always new vendors waiting to sell to an importing country that has quarantined a foreign supplier due to an outbreak of disease.

A few selected examples of imported disease reveal valid reasons for such international quarantines. In 1843 a ship's cow introduced contagious bovine pleuropneumonia into the United States. Scrapie was brought from the British

Isles via Canada (Hagan 1958). Movement of U.S. troops with their food, equipment, and supplies during and after World War II has been blamed for dissemination of hog cholera virus (Todd 1958). More recently, contagious equine metritis was imported into the United States with stallions from France (Holden 1978). It also should be noted that quarantines designed to exclude specific pathogens can keep out other pathogens as well. When Canada embargoed U.S. pork in the 1950s because of vesicular exanthema of swine, there was a reduction in hog cholera (Cockrill 1963).

All these incidents illustrate that until important pathogens have been eradicated, nations have only two choices: share diseases or try to maintain effective quarantine measures.

Effective regulatory legislation, whether dealing with quarantines or other health problems, must provide clear authority and must assign responsibility for enforcement to only one agency. An example of not following these precepts was the 1909 U.S. statute requiring importers of wild animals or birds to obtain an import permit from the Department of the Interior. However, that department was not given the discretion to withhold the permit, effectively emasculating authority to prevent entry. Furthermore, this same statute gave the Treasury Department the authority for making regulations to enforce the provisions of this statute. To exacerbate the situation, four separate federal departments (Interior; Treasury; Agriculture; and Health, Education, and Welfare) could require separate permits to import one wild animal (Pinkus 1968).

Strict preentry quarantine, first on the premises of the suppliers and then at the port of embarkation (with the exclusion of all animals in a group if there is even one infected animal) can be very effective, especially if combined with repeated laboratory testing. If a group is to be denied entry, this should be done as early as possible. The quarantine period must exceed the incubation periods for the major diseases of concern, and total faith in the quarantining agency is implicit in this technique.

Export quarantine facilities should be used exclusively for animals destined for exit and should be fully equipped with restraint facilities, communications, and utilities; easily cleanable; well drained; free of significant arthropod vectors; at least 200 meters from other livestock; convenient to transport; and protected by a security fence. All illnesses and deaths during quarantine should be investigated and the cause verified. Arthropod problems often can be minimized by prudent selection of the quarantine season (i.e., cold weather), plus use of proper insecticide sprays and dips.

Quarantine stations at the port of entry should meet the same specifications in addition to having facilities for treatment and necropsy and access to an incinerator. Quarantined import stock should be maintained in close contact with susceptible sentinel animals, and the facilities should operate on an all-in all-out basis. Sentinel animals play a unique role but they must be of unquestionable susceptibility, in adequate numbers, and be in close contact with the import animals for a sufficient time so that transmission is probable if the agent is present. Animals imported for slaughter must be maintained separately.

Isolation at the recipient farm in lieu of entry quarantine presents special problems, since producers with new animals understandably have an almost irresistible urge to show them off and put them to use.

# 8

# General Surveillance and Prevention of Spread

RISK REDUCTION through imposition of import control measures is a matter of degree rather than of absolutes; thus, some pathogen will breach the controls somewhere, sometime. There are also uncontrollable risk factors: wild species, including migratory birds; smuggling across national boundaries, an activity existing since the first ruler set up the first border control system. No system of barriers can prevent all introduction of disease; a system of surveillance and prevention of further spread is needed as a secondary defense.

## General Surveillance

Surveillance, in English, is derived from French words meaning "to watch over." As applied to national disease control, surveillance means a relatively specific or close watch. Although compulsory disease reporting dates back to 1729 in Prussia (Todd 1949), such scrutiny over all diseases has not been accomplished to date in medical history. Unless one adopts the convenient sham of requiring all disease to be reported and then proclaims the absence of reports as valid evidence of freedom from disease, a more meaningful method for ongoing surveillance of some type must be found.

Many countries publish a list of notifiable, reportable, or scheduled diseases—a relatively short list of those diseases felt to be of prime national importance. Because the list is limited to those few diseases generally recognized as unusually dangerous, the legal requirement that these be reported to animal health authorities is accepted as essential for the general welfare and becomes operationally practical.

A proper national or state surveillance system for notifiable diseases requires more than just case reporting; the system must call for the prompt follow-up investigation of reports within a time frame keyed to the urgency demanded. Without investigation, even a limited list of dangerous diseases requiring reporting is of little value in preventing the spread of disease. If funds and personnel permit, a most valuable adjunct is to combine the role of investigator and diagnostic consultant; thus practitioners can call on the con-trol agency for diagnostic consultation without losing face or violating client confidence. In return, the agency receives immediate, on-the-spot data concerning diagnostic dilemmas that could indicate the presence of a newly introduced agent or a novel manifestation of an old pathogen; either event would be of concern to a disease control agency. Also, agencies should provide laboratory support for the diagnosis of those diseases deemed reportable (Schnurrenberger and Hubbert 1981).

Because the resources required to maintain such a surveillance system are extensive, any list of notifiable diseases must be kept short if it is to function effectively. Therefore, governments often have a list of additional reportable diseases—those of lesser threat but still important to the public. Reports of these diseases are required or solicited from practitioners or other observers to give some indication of the location and frequency of occurrence of the diseases. Since reports from this secondary list may not call for follow-up investigation or regulatory action, reporting may be periodic rather than immediate. Accuracy of diagnosis is often a matter of clinical opinion unless accompanied by laboratory work, and case histories are usually sketchy and epidemiologic data lacking.

Because of the limited amount of proved information, general disease reporting systems do not provide the type of surveillance, including follow-up investigation, that results in limiting disease spread. It must be understood that these reporting systems are not designed for this purpose and information received must be kept in proper perspective. These systems only indicate what may be happening and are generally useful to practitioners, health protection agencies, and other interested groups for this purpose. Much of the national and international data on disease occurrence comes from these periodic reporting systems.

If expense is no object, active surveillance through field or laboratory examination of a structured sample of a population provides excellent information. Cost is the limiting factor. Collecting accurate information is always expensive; consequently, active surveillance is usually reserved for a campaign against a specific disease, and passive techniques are employed for general surveillance covering an array of diseases. Soper (1963) used the phrase "threshold of visibility," levels below which the mode of transmission cannot be detected with usual methods of surveillance, however, such thresholds often can be lowered through enhanced surveillance.

Surveillance, properly conducted, is an expensive, time consuming activity but not an end unto itself. It is rather a tool to be used in disease prevention, control, or eradication (Steele 1975). If the end result is to be justifiable in terms of time and money expended, the first decisions must be what information is needed, why it is needed, and how it will be used.

When the primary objective, to locate an agent by time and place and follow it through the population of concern, is achieved, the information acquired can be used in a variety of ways.

1. To aid in clinical diagnosis by knowing what diseases are present in an area.
2. To aid in informed program planning.
3. To provide baseline data for evaluating program progress.
4. To provide a warning of changes in the prevalence of diseases.
5. To permit an assessment of the impact of environmental changes (increased schistosomiasis after construction of Egypt's Aswan Dam), husbandry changes (decreased trichinosis following enforced cooking of garbage fed to hogs), social changes (increased hepatitis B with growth of the drug culture), and technological changes (appearance of Marburg disease with advances in tissue culture and vaccine production).

Further benefits accrue with closer surveillance and investigation of outbreaks.

6. A definition of high-risk groups in order to target control work.
7. A disclosure of vaccine problems (low egg passage–induced rabies in cattle, cats, and dogs).
8. The detection of sources of infection (airline garbage in African swine fever).
9. The assistance in vaccine production (typing isolates of FMD and human influenza virus).
10. The identification of factors favoring spread (rainfall, herd or flock management, reservoirs, vectors).
11. The identification of newly introduced disease agents.

**CLINICAL AND LABORATORY OBSERVATION.** The first phase of surveillance, observation, includes a variety of clinical and laboratory techniques. Good clinical observation depends on the sensitivity, training, and experience of the observer as well as his knowledge of the normal and the abnormal, including familiarity with the individual or group, lengthy observation without disturbing those observed, and a flexible concept of what the abnormal may be. From personal observation by one of the authors (Wise), it can be stated that the final three cases of vesicular exanthema of swine in the United States were so mild clinically that experienced vesicular disease diagnosticians could not readily identify affected swine by clinical observation alone. During their hog cholera eradication programs, Canada, Great Britain, Australia, and the United States found that many proven field cases did not fit the previously standard textbook patterns of an acute, highly fatal disease.

Significant support for disease surveillance is provided by diagnostic laboratories, and laboratory reports should be integrated into any surveillance system.

Laboratory observation is valuable for confirmation of clinical findings as well as for serologic survey or screening programs when there is a low case:infection ratio. The brucellosis ring test for dairy herds is a good example, as is the blood testing of market cattle in the United States to identify suspect or reactor animals and trace them to their herd of origin. These market cattle identification (MCI) sera are not random samples of the cattle population; however, for the purposes of brucellosis surveillance, it is desirable to obtain a biased sample from animals culled for reasons such as age or clinical signs of disease. On the other hand when using this system, it has been shown that low culling rates, small herd sizes, low infection rates, and low sample collection rates decrease the probability of finding infected herds.

In spite of the difficulties encountered (identification, record keeping, etc.), there is no doubt that the MCI program is a valuable surveillance tool for brucellosis in the United States. The program also has potential use in epidemiologic surveillance of other cattle diseases, including tuberculosis, and has been used by some states in the study of anaplasmosis, bluetongue, and bovine leukosis. The Australian system uses tail tags rather than back tags and includes color as another useful facet. When blue tags are used rather than white tags, individual animals can be identified rather than just the farm of origin. In these instances, facts relevant to the individual animals can be returned to the owner as an aid in making management decisions.

Laboratory-based surveillance programs tend to cost more than clinical surveillance alone. As with clinical surveillance, unless the sample approaches 100% of the animals involved or has been selected by statistically sound methods, laboratory results will be biased and cannot be used to determine incidence or prevalence. However, they can indicate trends if records are maintained for an adequate time and submission and examination practices remain constant. The records should be examined carefully for bias before drawing conclusions (Christiansen 1979).

If spot testing is used to project prevalence in an area, sampling must be conducted carefully to avoid drawing erroneous conclusions. The sample tested should be selected either by statistically random techniques or by concentrating on high-risk segments of the population, remembering that field personnel have a tendency to collect samples from the easiest spot, not necessarily the most meaningful one. Another caveat is that later samples should be from different portions of the population so that, given sufficient time, all members will be tested.

The telltale pockmarks of smallpox provided yet another method for conducting surveillance: predetermined sampling of populations and calculation of age-specific pock rates (Brilliant and Hodakevic 1978). This method is not suitable for all diseases, but it is applicable to those where vaccination leaves a distinctive scar or where pathognomonic lesions are visible in animals slaughtered for food. A combination of this lesion detection method and sequential sampling is used for malaria where splenomegaly detection is rapid and economical. When splenomegaly is detected, a confirmatory blood smear is collected.

**DATA COLLECTION.** The second phase of surveillance is data collection, which presents a problem that has not been solved over large areas or long periods of time. Bridging the gap between true occurrence and numbers appearing on official records requires an awareness of the "iceberg phenomenon," alluding to the small portion of an iceberg visible above the water. An example is the smallpox program in India. The state of Uttar Pradesh, with a population of 90 million, had regularly been reporting from 100 to 300 cases of smallpox per week. The first one-week search found more than 7000 cases, and a later assessment showed that only half of the villages officially reported as having been searched had actually been visited (Henderson 1976).

Another demonstration of reporting discrepancies is a chorioptic scabies project where 1200 cases were disclosed in the first 6 months compared with 2 cases reported in the preceding 5 years (McCallon 1973).

Discrepancies in occurrence and those actually reported cannot be ignored by health protection agencies, particularly in programs that depend heavily on initial reports of apparent disease based on clinical observation. To assume that reports received represent all disease that occurred is to invite failure. A proven method of attacking this problem is to promote reporting of *any* evidence, even remote suspicion, of the disease in question—the emphasis being on a large volume of suspicious reports, each of which is subsequently investigated in depth. The key to reducing the unseen portion of the iceberg is to aim for a wide ratio between suspicious reports and those eventually confirmed rather than emphasizing only the confirmed cases. During the hog cholera eradication program in Great Britain, animal health authorities sought a 10:1, suspect:confirm ratio in order to have some confidence that all actual hog cholera was being found. In the United States the initial goal of 10:1 reached 131:1 in 1976, the last year in which hog cholera was found. The same concept has been an important aspect of field surveillance in the screwworm program in the United States and Mexico. Livestock owners are asked to submit to the laboratory all fly larvae found in wounds, rather than deciding in the field which are actually screwworms. The number of negative reports indicates the intensity of owner cooperation and the effectiveness of those promoting reporting. A similar situation occurs when animal owners and veterinarians are asked to report all suspected vesicular conditions during an outbreak of a specific vesicular disease.

An optimal reporting program should be complete, accurate, prompt, detailed, and possess denominator data. However, errors and losses do result from subclinical infections, unobserved cases, misdiagnoses, unreported diagnoses, losses during relay to the tabulating agency, and error in tabulation. Terminology also may be a problem. In the same region, a disease may be known by different names, or similar syndromes involving separate causes may bear the same name. A worldwide attempt has been made to standardize terms in veterinary medicine (National Cancer Institute 1969), including the acronyms SVNDO (Standard Veterinary Nomenclature of Diseases and Operations), SNOP (Standard Nomenclature of Pathology), ICCDA (International Classification of Causes of Diseases and Accidents), and VMDP (Veterinary Medical Data Program). Uniform definitions and a system of disease classification are prerequisite to advancing scientific knowledge (Hutton 1975).

One difficulty with some of these systems is the large number of codes for conditions that are nearly similar clinically, defeating efforts to achieve consistency when many clinicians and coders are involved. The caliber of these personnel is vital to the success of the system, for a surveillance system is only as reliable as the source of its data. However, depending on its use, diagnostic accuracy is less important on a regional basis as long as it is consistent. Mussman et al. (1979) pointed out that, especially in developing countries, there is a tendency to place the responsibility for diagnosis and reporting on the least technically qualified people, who also lack personnel, transportation, and communication. Their reports, however, often form the data on which policies and programs are formed.

Another difficulty is the opinions that arise regarding the cause of a disease; these opinions can be avoided by coding for clinical signs rather than diagnoses (Leech 1979). However, this combines diseases with different epidemiologic patterns. Also, changes in diagnostic criteria, terminology, or reporting procedures result in situations where data cannot be compared over time, precluding analysis of secular trends. For this reason a precise definition of what constitutes a case is essential to a sophisticated surveillance effort. This becomes vastly more important as an agent nears extinction, for accurate case determination is essential at that time.

As mentioned earlier, a common approach to reporting can center on a published list of reportable diseases under government authority. This approach is particularly applicable in areas that are well covered by private practitioners. However, a recent study of the frequency of required reporting of selected zoonoses in the United States found that (1) public health agencies required reporting of more zoonoses than animal health agencies, (2) there was no consistency between states, and (3) there was no coordination between the two agencies within a state (Schnurrenberger and Hubbert 1980). This suggests that there is no real uniformity in the method of deciding which diseases should be reported.

Most disease-reporting programs in human medicine are reinforced by required reports of births and deaths, which are often supplemented by a periodic, detailed census, providing accurate data on population characteristics such as age, race, and sex. This type of information is rarely available for nonhuman populations.

Another surveillance method for selected chronic diseases is the use of registries, where each case is registered as a distinct entity, then followed closely. This is an old established system in public health agencies for diseases such as typhoid, tuberculosis and cancer, but it is an uncommon practice in nonhuman species.

In animal health work, another approach is to select certain veterinary practices or specific herds for surveillance efforts and limit data collection to these practices or premises except for emergency situations such as the introduction of an exotic disease. This usually provides more complete and accurate data since the participants are more highly motivated. However, the number of participants is usually so limited that it is difficult to extrapolate the data to a broader population.

The Danes have developed a successful nationwide surveillance system combining traceback and abattoir inspection, which was organized in 1964 through a national farmers' cooperative; it now includes 80% of their bacon pigs. The pigs receive a backslap tattoo and are shipped directly to an abattoir under veterinary inspection where diagnoses are made under a uniform nomenclature. Data such as herd of origin, weight class, sex, diagnosis, abattoir, and week of slaughter are encoded in a central computer. Since the number of pigs slaughtered coincides quite well with herd size, denominator data can be approximated, allowing for the evaluation of seasonal and geographic trends, interherd variation by housing and management, plus evaluation of specific pathogen-free herds. It is, however, limited to diseases with severe lesions and underestimates conditions with high mortality, for many of these pigs never reach market (Willeberg 1979).

Without employing the sophisticated traceback, computer assistance, and denominator data of the Danish system, New Zealand has utilized abattoir data for prevalence surveys on bovine brucellosis, Johne's disease, leptospirosis, pseudorabies, enzootic pneumonia, and bovine adenocarcinoma (Christiansen and Hellstorm 1979). Data on 18 diseases are compiled from all 73 abattoirs and rates are calculated on the basis of species, disease, region, and month. Although there are some disadvantages (subclinical conditions, seasonal slaughter, diagnosis on gross morphology only), the system uses existing specimens, labor, and inspection systems.

Transmission of initial reports is usually limited to mail, telephone, or cable, with couriers utilized only in remote areas when laboratory samples are submitted with the report, or when a laboratory sample, if carelessly handled or lost, may cause disease in a previously clean area. Collection of reports is usually more effective if it is government financed and if reminders are sent out for each collecting period. Such periods should be no longer than 1 month, except for emergencies, as inaccuracies increase as the period lengthens, and frequent collection becomes tedious for the reporter, diminishing cooperation. However, it is vital that emergencies be recognized as they arise and that they are reported by the most expeditious means available. A collecting agency consolidates the reports into a single composite through hand tabulation or computer techniques.

Evaluation of the consolidated reports, on the other hand, is the reason surveillance programs exist and should not be neglected. It requires a background in epidemiology, clinical medicine, and preventive medicine; experience and judgment; and attentiveness through the periods of tedium when analyzing routine data in order to quickly see the appearance, usually unexpected, of significant change.

Modern computer techniques can be an invaluable aid. Ray (1980) observed that while the files of the USDA Brucellosis Eradication Program contained invaluable epidemiologic information, the vast majority of it was unavailable for program management because retrieval would require manual effort. Complete records are essential but so is accessibility. The Australians have made a major stride toward developing an accessible system in the Australian National Animal Disease Information System, ANADIS (Roe 1979): each regional laboratory updates its computer records daily with the brucellosis test results then mails the magnetic disks to national headquarters weekly. Field veterinarians can access the laboratory computer by telephone and alter the test interpretation if indicated epidemiologically. This decentralized system provides state-to-state flexibility keyed to field needs, furnishes immediate access to up-to-the-minute records, eliminates many clerical errors, identifies emerging problems early, permits study of factors affecting progress, improves cost effectiveness, provides parameter values for simulation models, and allows extrapolation for program predictions.

The information collected and analyzed should be disseminated to participants, control authorities, and other groups of interest in a meaningful, timely, and understandable form. Participants will not continue to operate if uninformed; they need the returns to encourage continued participation. For animal disease reports, for example, the Food and Agriculture Organization, the World Health Organization, and the International Office of Epizootics annually combine resources to publish the Animal Health Yearbook.

It is essential that dissemination of information includes an accurate interpretation so that the data can be perceived in proper perspective by the recipients, especially for the laity (general public, livestock industry, or news media), who seldom are skilled in interpreting such data. Even with objective analysis accompanying the data, misinterpretations can be made. Without analysis, mountains of misinformation may be constructed on a molehill of basic facts.

Population cycles can influence the effectiveness of surveillance programs. For example, programs centering around terminal markets may yield excellent results when herds are being liquidated, as in drought periods or times of low profitability, but will be poor sources during a herd build-up stage. This discrepancy can be partially countered by surveillance based on movements between farms.

## Prevention of Spread

All reports of suspicious or unusual disease conditions should be promptly investigated. While many will be false alarms, one case of serious disease reported and investigated promptly may save a costly campaign. There may be reluctance to report the possibility of a foreign disease with clinical similarities to a native disease; for example, African swine fever and hog cholera or FMD and vesicular stomatitis. Clinicians, in particular, may be reluctant to undergo the perceived embarrassment of a misdiagnosis. In actuality, clinicians who do make such reports are demonstrating a superior sense of professional and public responsibility and should be recognized accordingly.

No modern health protection agency would attempt a control or eradication program against a specific disease agent without including a strong component devoted to public education. No regulatory measure aimed at preventing disease spread will be effective unless the affected public understands the reasons for the actions and the purposes they serve. With an informed public, the common preventive measures of health certification, isolation, quarantine, and vaccination will be understood as meeting a valid public purpose, assuming, of course, that credibility is maintained by imposing only those restrictions that have a valid public purpose.

Health certification is one general preventive technique required in many countries for animals moving from one premises to another, or through markets or other buying and selling points. Given a sufficient number of competent health inspection personnel strategically located at trade routes and centers, it provides worthwhile public protection in preventing spread of many disease agents and insurance against deception for prospective purchasers. Public confidence in the procedure is necessary and can be maintained if the system is practical (i.e., if it is timely and not burdened with excessive paper-shuffling requirements) and is perceived as free from fraud or deception.

Although the terms isolation and quarantine often are used interchangeably, isolation should be used when referring to infected animals, usually active cases, and quarantine when dealing with animals that are susceptible or of unknown status. In either instance, the objective is to reduce interanimal contacts and inhibit the transmission of pathogens. These techniques are of limited benefit with agents that are transmitted by indirect routes, unless vehicles and vectors are controlled along with the animal hosts. Controls on movement may be extended to include cleaning and disinfection stations at important travel hubs and may even include establishing livestock-free buffer zones around infected areas.

General quarantines, while perhaps of some value for public relations purposes, are expensive and not easy to administer effectively. Cost assessment should be a part of training exercises in order to instill the realization that even a local quarantine is costly to livestock producers and others in the processing and marketing chain. It is also important that quarantines, either general or restricted, not be issued without stating the conditions that, if met, will result in the quarantine release. Without this step, any quarantine eventually will be ignored and will be an embarrassment to the issuing agency. Good quarantine policy requires a system for checking on compliance. A general quarantine over a wide area against whole classes of animals usually rules out the practicality of good quarantine inspection. When narrowed to a more specific target that involves a minority group of producers who may threaten the majority, a general quarantine is useful in general disease prevention.

An example of specific targeting would be a general quarantine of the few swine producers that feed their livestock swill or garbage. Scientifically, there is no question that this practice is potentially dangerous and has repeatedly led to spread of disease. Permanent quarantine and inspection of such premises, with movement under permit and only directly to slaughter, is a valuable addition to other preventive measures, such as required heat-treating of food waste before it is fed to swine.

It must be emphasized again, however, that preventing the spread of disease, in a general sense, is primarily dependent on an educated public that knows why it is profitable to maintain good environmental sanitation and nutrition, reduce contact with potentially risky populations or individuals, and use immunizing agents to assist in maintaining general health.

# 9
## Understanding Laboratory and Sampling Processes

DETECTION OF DISEASE AGENTS is increasingly dependent upon laboratory results, which have grown with the application of new microbiologic and immunologic methods. It is essential that these results are dependable and only come from laboratories of proven capability. This often necessitates a laboratory or technician certification system, complete with training, facility inspection, reagent quality control, submission of unknowns, and verification of acceptability.

This certification hierarchy assumes the existence of at least one reference laboratory with unimpeachable credentials that is available for consultation with developing laboratories and provides both the initial training and follow-up support services. The final system may consist of a sophisticated, certified central laboratory with satellites performing only service functions such as separating sera and shipping specimens to the central laboratory. At the other end of the scale is a central facility that is merely one among equals, being denoted central only because of its propinquity to the program's administrative leader. Between these extremes lie endless potential variations with the final organizational structure based on such factors as workload, communication and transportation systems, test sophistication, urgency of results for program decisions, livestock distribution, personnel capabilities, funding, political demands, and the type of problem being solved. To prevent unethical practices in eradication programs, it may be necessary to prohibit testing by any noncertified laboratories to preclude screening specimens and removing positives before they are submitted for official testing.

The sensitivity of the laboratory methods and the kinds of disease agents that can be detected are far different from what they were only a few years ago.

This chapter, with the exception of the last subsection (Significance of Sampling), was prepared by Dr. Robert Hanson, Professor of Veterinary Science, University of Wisconsin.

However, the detection of new agents and the surveillance of those already present is a more complex process than merely determining the presence or absence of a disease agent or antibody in a sample presented to the laboratory. Detection is a four step process: (1) questioning (what information is needed?), (2) sampling (what procedure should be used?), (3) testing (what method is appropriate?), and (4) interpreting (how are the results to be interpreted and used?).

Laboratory tests may answer two kinds of questions: qualitative, whether the sample test is reactive, and quantitative, the degree of reactivity (e.g., the height of titer or number of organisms). Both answers are subject to many qualifications. Depending on the disease, reactor status may mean that the individual is a carrier or, conversely, once was infected and now is free of infection. The magnitude of response or serologic titer that indicates resistance to one disease agent may indicate susceptibility to another.

## Evolution of Diagnostic Tests

Microbiologists and immunologists have devised a great variety of tests to obtain answers to questions concerning the state of infection and resistance to disease. These tests differ in sensitivity, accuracy, time needed for completion, and cost. Particular efforts must be made to determine if a given test is appropriate for answering a specific question.

**DEVELOPMENT OF TESTS.** Development of a given test starts in the laboratory with the application of an idea, such as using a Vero cell culture to isolate a respiratory virus from nasal swabs or a system for measuring the quantity of neutralizing antibodies in serum to determine whether there has been exposure to a disease agent. In either situation many variables must be understood if the test is to be useful.

To measure antibodies, a suitable indicator must be found in which a regular overt response is obtained (such as the development of plaques in a cell culture or death of an intracerebrally inoculated mouse). Quantitative (dilution of virus and serum) and temporal (time allowed for interaction) relationships of test reagents must then be established.

Using an indicator that works when the constituents are controlled is only the first step. In order to interpret the results, the investigator must know how soon neutralizing antibodies are developed following infection and how long this responsiveness is retained after recovery. In some diseases, antibodies are retained for years, possibly for life, whereas for others the response is temporary, sometimes disappearing in a few weeks. The investigator also needs to know whether the disease agent is eliminated before antibody develops or whether it persists. Obviously, a serologic test for those few diseases in which the disease agent may persist even after the antibody becomes undetectable would be of limited use in a regulatory program.

The answers to these questions must be determined for each species affected by the disease agent, as each may be unique: different age groups may respond with enough difference to merit comparison before conclusions are drawn from the tests. In young animals, antibodies may have been transferred from their mothers during their first weeks of life and do not signify an active infection. The effect of vaccine prophylaxis and antibiotic therapy on serologic response must be known.

**DETERMINATION OF SENSITIVITY AND SPECIFICITY.** The sensitivity and specificity of a new test can be determined by using experimental data to fill the cells A, B, C, and D in Table 9.1. A perfect test would have all results in A (truly infected and test positive) or D (not infected and test negative), with none in B (not infected but test positive) or C (truly infected but test negative). Few tests fit this pattern perfectly. The calculations use the following formulas: sensitivity $= A/(A+C)$ and specificity $= D/(D+B)$.

**Table 9.1. Data cells for determining sensitivity and specificity of tests**

| Reaction | Infected | Not Infected |
|---|---|---|
| Positive | A | B |
| Negative | C | D |

To illustrate the impact of sensitivity, take a hypothetical herd of 1000 cattle, 50 of which are infected with a disease that has a transmission rate of 10% per month. One month also is the interval between herd tests; all reactors are removed at each test period. Assuming we test the herd with a test that is 100% sensitive and 100% specific, our first test will detect all 50 infected cattle but none of the uninfected cattle will react. The herd is cleaned of infection in a single test cycle, leaving the owner with 950 healthy cattle.

However, if we had used a test that was 100% sensitive but only 50% specific, the results would have differed markedly. The first test still would have removed all 50 infected animals but also would have falsely declared 475 noninfected cattle as reactors (specificity $= D/[D + B]$ so 50% $= D/950$, therefore $D = 475$). This would leave the owner with a healthy herd but only 475 cattle and a strong distaste for the program.

If we had used a test with 90% sensitivity and 90% specificity (not totally unrealistic characteristics), the first test would have removed 140 cattle (45 of the 50 infected plus 95 noninfected). We would have to assume that the 5 remaining carriers would infect 1 new animal during the next month, so there would be 6 infected and 854 noninfected cattle present for the second test. Five infected (90% of 6 = 5.4) and 85 noninfected cattle (90% = 768.6/854) would be removed with this test, leaving 1 and 769 respectively. There would be no new infections (10% of 1 = 0.1), and the third test should detect the remaining infected animal leaving a clean herd. The third test also would remove 77 healthy animals (90% = 692.1/769), leaving the farmer with a healthy herd of 692 cattle and the expense of gathering his cattle three times for testing. The government would fund their portion of collecting and testing 2630 samples (1000 + 860 + 770) plus an indemnity for 308 cattle.

An even worse situation would arise if the test was 10% sensitive and 100% specific. The first test would remove only 5 infected cattle, leaving 45 carriers that would produce 5 new infections by the second test. This would be repeated at each test cycle with new infections occurring as rapidly as reactors were detected, resulting in a constant number of infected animals while the number of uninfected animals decreased slowly until the entire herd had been depleted. The agent and herd would be eradicated simultaneously.

As eradication nears, it may be wise to use the most sensitive test for screening purposes, even if specificity is sacrificed for that sensitivity. Sera that react to the screening test are then subjected to more specific tests and the herds are investigated epidemiologically to arrive at the final diagnosis.

**FIELD EVALUATION.** After the validity and meaning of a test have been established under experimental conditions, they should be tried in the field. Samples from a genetically diverse population, collected and handled under a variety of environmental conditions, may reflect a considerable variation in the sensitivity and specificity of a test. Geographic differences can cause marked variations; e.g., tuberculin testing. At this point, the time and cost to conduct the test must be carefully evaluated: automation may reduce time and labor costs; conversion from large test tubes to small wells in a microtiter plate may reduce the volume of reagents needed, thus reduce cost; or the test may even be adapted for field use, such as the brucellosis and anaplasmosis card tests or the pullorum agglutination test. When changes are made, however, test attributes may be altered. The old and new procedure should be carried out in parallel until it is established that the change does not produce undesirable differences in sensitivity or specificity.

Interpretation is facilitated by having available field data on the specimens that were submitted; diagnostic laboratories request that historical and clinical data accompany all specimens. However, final diagnosis is the responsibility of the clinician in charge, or the director of a disease program.

Tests designed for field use address special problems and unique needs. They provide a convenience that is especially appreciated in extensive operations where gathering and confining livestock presents special problems and expenses. They negate the need for permanent identification and, since the determination of reactor status can be made immediately, there is no need to regather entire herds to search for and remove the few reactors. Penside tests also serve a valuable public relations purpose; the owner can see the test results firsthand.

Field tests have special requirements: they must utilize fluids or tissues that can be collected in the field without special processing, such as heat inactivation; they must not require bulky or sensitive equipment or be rendered inaccurate by dust, rain, or other adverse conditions.

There is an extraordinary opportunity for abuse of field tests if unscrupulous individuals obtain access to test materials. The tests lend themselves to screening use so that reactor animals can be excluded from official tests or, even worse, sold to unsuspecting buyers without official tests.

## Interpretation of Diagnostic Tests

**POSITIVES.** The usual question asked of laboratory staff is, "Is it positive?" The answer depends on the program objective. Isolation of an agent does not necessarily mean that the agent is inducing disease or detection of antigen that the agent possessing that antigen is still infective. Detection of antibody does not tell whether the infection was recent or not, whether the individual is a carrier, or whether the carrier has recovered and is resistant or susceptible to reinfection.

If a question is asked, a test to answer the question is designed or employed and the results evaluated. The program officials then decide whether the results should be considered positive. If an exotic agent is invading a new region, only isolation of the agent will be an acceptable positive, whereas within a diseased area, demonstration of reactor status by any method is often sufficient. This does not mean eradication efforts will be delayed until an agent has been isolated and unquestionably identified. Preliminary investigation and quarantine may be instituted at the earliest hint, even before laboratory specimens are collected.

**FALSE POSITIVES.** False positives appear in most tests at a certain and usually low frequency. Some appear only at the presumptive stage, disappearing when the confirmatory test is applied. Isolation of a hemagglutinating agent lethal to chicken embryos can mean something other than Newcastle disease virus; a confirmatory antigen identity test determines if it truly is Newcastle disease virus.

False positives in serologic tests sometimes are more difficult to detect. While most nonspecific reactive substances in serum are more heat labile than true antibody and more sensitive to certain other treatments, there are exceptions. On occasion, investigators have to demonstrate that the resistant neutralizing substance, for example for influenza in calves, was not in the globulin fraction of the serum where true antibody is found and was therefore nonspecific (this is impractical as a routine procedure).

An alternative method of recognizing nonspecific reactors (false positives) has been used in some large serum surveys. An extensive study of the sheep population of Tierra del Fuego was conducted by a United States-Argentine commission with the British and Chilean governments to determine if the island was free of foot-and-mouth disease virus. It was suspected that even if no true antibodies were found there would be nonspecific reactors that would cloud the status of the islands. Therefore, sera were also obtained from a genetically similar sheep population in New Zealand, a country also in the Antipodes, whose freedom from foot-and-mouth disease has never been questioned. A very low frequency of reactors was found in the New Zealand sheep and a similar rate occurred in the sheep from Tierra del Fuego. Also, and in spite of the old dictum that nonspecific reactors are not serotype specific, most were either Type A or Type O and few reacted to both antigenic types. A similar number of reactors was found in later studies conducted on sera from cattle in the United States. Numerous examples of such cross-reactive antigens have been documented for bacteria and other viruses.

Nonspecific reactors not only can cause confusion in general surveys but can be damaging in specific control or eradication programs, particularly when infection has been reduced to a low level. Obviously, if the problem is not recognized, no end point in reactors will ever be reached if diagnosis is solely dependent on laboratory results.

**NEGATIVES.** Finding a negative may be just as important as finding a positive. However, a negative test does not necessarily mean the pathogen is not or was not present; it also can mean that the test was insensitive. In addition, a true negative test in a single animal may not reflect the status of the herd. Before reporting a negative finding, one needs to determine the sensitivity of the test and the adequacy of the sampling procedure.

From a regulatory point of view, demonstrating the negative status of a herd is important in four situations: (1) evaluating progress in a control or eradication campaign, (2) establishing the success of an eradication program in an area to be freed from quarantine, (3) establishing the suitability of animals to be imported, and (4) certifying the specific pathogen-free status of animals used for certain purposes. In fact, being able to demonstrate the absence of a disease or pathogen is the goal of most prevention, control, and eradication programs.

Establishing a valid negative test depends on the sensitivity of the test and the nature of the disease. Isolation of some bacteria and viruses is relatively simple because the culture system is sensitive and, if an individual is infected, the agent will almost invariably be found at certain sites. Isolation of other bacteria or viruses is difficult because a sensitive culture system is not available; the agent either is not regularly present, is hidden at an inaccessible site, or is bound in some fashion that requires special procedures for demonstration; or isolation takes a very long time. A negative test for the first group of agents has considerable significance but it may have little meaning for the second group.

Failure to detect antibody in an animal is meaningful for those diseases in which a carrier state is always associated with antibody, as well as those diseases in which persistent antibody titers follow full recovery. It is of no value for pathogens that induce a transient antibody response followed by complete recovery, that have persistent or intermittent carriers after the antibody response disappears, or that induce no antibody at all.

Assuming that one has a valid test, a quarantine can be initiated for an appropriate period, with samples taken at the beginning and end of the period. A negative test at both samplings usually clears that individual or group.

**FALSE NEGATIVES.** Because of the extreme variability inherent in biological systems (including those of the agent, host, and the test itself), no test is 100% accurate. There is always the potential for a false positive or a false negative result. This potential for error means there will be situations where clinical and epidemiologic findings conflict with laboratory results, creating a possible problem for the veterinarian who is responsible for the final diagnostic decision. This decision obviously is influenced heavily by the relative strengths of the evidence from the three areas, but it may hinge on the cost of an erroneous positive diagnosis (unnecessarily activating an alarm system) versus a false negative (missing an infection).

These same cost considerations come into play when deciding on the titer that will be considered reactive, for the titer determines whether the test interpretation will favor sensitivity or specificity (these factors are reciprocal, as one increases the other decreases). To illustrate, if the titer that is considered reactive is raised from 1:100 to 1:200, the test effectively becomes more specific (there will be fewer false positives) but less sensitive (more false negatives, more missed infections). As a result, as the prevalence decreases and eradication nears, the titer designating official reactors should be lowered. Indeed, this will result in condemnation of some uninfected animals through the decreased specificity, but the increased sensitivity will mean fewer infected animals go undetected.

In the final stages of eradication programs it is prudent to request that subordinate laboratories submit all positive specimens and a randomly selected percentage (5–10% would be desirable) of their negative specimens to the reference laboratory for confirmation. The reason for this was stated by Biberstein et al. (1961).

> It is a truism that the last residue of infection in a population behaves more erratically in regard to ordinary diagnostic reactions than does a group where no check has ever been applied to the infection previously.

This has been the experience in all situations where an infectious disease has been brought under control as in the case of bovine tuberculosis and human syphilis and the problem of false tests had assumed proportions it never had when the infections were widespread.

It is probable that the perceived behavioral differences really represent increased awareness of the total clinical spectrum produced by an agent and relative elimination of the pathogen strains that produce "classic" disease.

**FORENSIC SIGNIFICANCE OF DIAGNOSIS.** In veterinary medicine, demonstrating the presence of carriers in a herd, flock, or shipment of animals will result in their devaluation and possibly in condemnation. Since test results sometimes will be contested, results should be defensible in a court of law. To stand challenge, the laboratory should observe the following practice:

1. The identity of the sample should be protected at all times as it moves through the laboratory; the sample must never be misplaced or put in an inappropriate place.

2. It must be determined that the protocol to be followed is acceptable to other laboratories as good practice.

3. The protocol to which the sample is subjected must be maintained in writing, and it must be followed.

4. Aliquots of the specimens should be preserved for retesting, if necessary.

5. It is important to establish a policy on retesting, how many times a specimen will be retested, and which results are acceptable. Be prepared to defend the policy.

6. Accurate records should be kept in laboratory log books, with entries dated and preferably signed or initialled by the observer.

7. Preserve the records.

To determine the accuracy of the work and quality of reagents being used, some laboratory directors periodically obtain coded positive and negative samples and have them processed as unknowns; serologists may exchange titered serum samples and antigen lots to cross-check procedures and materials. Protocols, equipment, and reagents have been improved as a result. These practices, which go beyond the standard positive and negative controls employed in many tests, strengthen the position of a laboratory when any of its results are presented in court.

## Significance of Sampling

Testing every animal in large populations is usually prohibitive in cost and may be logistically impossible. The next option is to test materials obtained from a representative group of animals, which requires a statistically valid, random sample.

A truly random sample of a large population (one that gives every individual an equal chance of being selected) presumes an exact knowledge of the population and the existence of an identification system. However, such a system seldom exists and, like testing every animal, is logistically complicated and costly. Therefore, random sampling of domestic animal populations is usually done on a herd basis with the herds randomly selected from a population that has first been stratified, usually on a geographic basis. An example would be to divide a region into districts (e.g., 10), subdivide the districts into areas (e.g., 10), and then select one area in each district for sampling. In the areas selected, either all the herds or a random sample are tested. This method is administratively and logistically manageable, as travel is reduced and education programs can be pinpointed to the participants.

Characteristics of the sample selected should be compared with those of the total population in the epidemiologically significant characteristics such as group (herd) size, age structure, and management styles (confined, free ranging, closed, or open). Sampling within the selected herds also must be random.

For convenience and economy the quality of the sample is sometimes sacrificed by resorting to collection at markets and abattoirs. Such a sample has advantages in achieving some program objectives, however, it is far too biased to permit projecting results to the total population and cannot yield accurate prevalence data.

Sample size is determined by the size of the acceptable error (the reverse of level of confidence), error being lowest with a large sample and largest with a small sample. Beal (1975a) shows that to achieve 99% confidence of detecting disease in a 1000-unit herd with a 2% disease level, 204 animals must be sampled. If only 90% confidence is desired in the same herd, sample size can be reduced to 108.

Another factor to take into account is the frequency with which reactors may be expected to occur in the population. Reactor rate is primarily an agent-determined characteristic, approaching 100% for some diseases and close to 1% for others. Obviously, a small sample (1 of every 50) would have a better chance of finding the first type of infection than would a large sample (1 of every 5) in finding the latter. Sampling tables are available that also take this factor into account.

A sample that has been properly selected, correctly identified, and carefully preserved also becomes a valuable legacy for future generations. Regardless of the original reason it was collected, such a bank can be used later when new tests are developed or disease interests change. The question always arises as to prevalence in years past, and serum and tissue banks can help provide the answers. Testing 3199 sera preserved from a 1974 hog cholera survey revealed only 0.56% positive for pseudorabies. A selected sample of 6907 swine sera collected in 1977 was 3.53% positive for pseudorabies, strongly suggesting that a marked increase in prevalence had occurred (Schnurrenberger 1978).

Sampling precautions also apply to specimens collected from individual animals. As specific examples, if organisms are distributed sporadically through an animal's feces, improper sampling might easily result in negative results. If such an animal is cultured repeatedly, the data could easily be misinterpreted as depicting intermittent shedding (Leech 1979).

# 10

# Observations on Vaccination

IMMUNOLOGY had its inception in the eighteenth century with the classic work of Jenner, followed in the nineteenth century by the work of Pasteur, Metchnikoff, Ehrlich, Von Behring, and others. New plateaus were reached in the middle of the twentieth century: an understanding of the nature of antigens emerged during the 1950s, of antibodies during the 1960s, and of cellular immunity in the 1970s. In the 1980s the "manufacture" of immunizing agents through recombinations of genetic material began.

This progress covered only about 200 years and has enabled improvements that prevent many infectious diseases that once killed millions of humans and their animals. It has become technologically feasible to develop safe and efficacious vaccines that are easily administered and offer long-term protection. As a result, vaccination programs can be carried out on a large scale, with the purpose of preventing overt clinical disease by preventing infection or limiting host response.

It is currently accepted that there are two aspects of the specific host defense system: (1) the humoral (antibody) system, which consists of B (bursa-dependent) lymphocytes and four immunoglobulin classes (IgG, IgM, IgA, and IgE), plus helper cells. To assist this system there are K (killer) cells, phagocytic cells, and effector molecules such as complement and properdine; and (2) the cell-mediated immune system, which consists of T (thymus-dependent) lymphocytes, macrophages, and a number of products of these cells called lymphokines and monokines. Available information suggests that vaccine protection is mediated primarily through humoral immunity and secondarily through cell-mediated immunity (CMI), particularly in situations where vaccination prevents infection, as with effective vaccination against such agents as hog cholera, rabies, and canine distemper. However, when vaccination protects against the development of clinical disease but not infection (leptospirosis and tetanus), then CMI and local antibody play important and perhaps primary roles in preventing disease.

The aim of a good vaccine is to elicit both cellular and humoral immune responses that will prevent infection, not just disease, for in disease the vaccinated animals may continue to transmit the pathogen. Another problem arises when the vaccine induces humoral antibody that interferes with diagnostic tests. This is especially important if there is a program to control or eradicate an agent and the program includes either serologic or intradermal testing. In these situations it may be impossible, or at least extremely difficult, to distinguish between a titer due to vaccination, denoting protection, and a titer caused by infection, signifying a possible source for others.

The primary function of an immune response is to protect a host against infectious agents. However, occasionally an immune response causes tissue damage or discomfort by producing an allergic reaction (atropy); responding to self-antigen with subsequent disease (autoimmunity); the immune cells becoming neoplastic (myeloma); or by the cells of the immune system failing to differentiate or function properly, resulting in an immunodeficiency disorder.

The term immune is used here in a broad sense, including both relative and absolute protection against disease; however, to be correct it should be used only in the absolute sense. Resistance is the proper term when speaking relatively and the overwhelming majority of our vaccination procedures induce only increased resistance, not total protection. Most vaccine protection can be overwhelmed when given a sufficiently severe exposure.

## Factors Influencing Host Defense Systems

Factors influencing a host defense system can affect immune response to a vaccine. Those to be considered in designing an effective vaccination program include (1) the immunosuppressive (blocking) effect of colostral antibody, (2) the other immune sera, (3) the nature of the vaccine, (4) the route of vaccination, (5) the age of the recipient, (6) the general nutritional condition of the recipient, (7) the concurrent infection, and (8) the drug treatments.

**COLOSTRAL ANTIBODY.** In many species, most, if not all, of the immunoglobulin in a newborn comes from absorption of colostrum shortly after birth. Following absorption from the gut, specific colostral antibodies have the ability to prevent most vaccine antigens from reaching the lymphocytes and macrophages, which are responsible for the genesis of active immunity. Therefore, the passively acquired antibody of colostral origin must drop to low levels before active immunization is possible. This period of uncertain response to vaccination may last as long as 14–16 weeks after birth. Heterotypic vaccines (e.g., measles virus for canine distemper) may circumvent this effect. High-titer vaccines (large antigenic doses) may be more effective in overcoming low levels of passive (colostral) antibody than low-titer vaccines. These methods are not absolute, however, and as it is extremely important that colostral antibody be available to protect neonates during the first few weeks of life, no attempt should be made to deprive newborn animals of colostrum.

**IMMUNE SERA.** Passive protection in the form of immune serum, hyperimmune serum, or gamma globulin has been described as the "miracle worker that isn't." One needs to understand the potential of these products and consider them for what they are. To be effective, they must contain high levels of antibody to the specific organism one wants to protect against. While immune serum or gamma globulin will be of little or no value after clinical signs of disease appear, in certain cases they will be effective if given immediately after exposure. Whether they protect against infection or just against clinical diseases depends on the agent involved.

It must be recognized that immune globulin can interfere with active immunization similar to the interference caused by colostral immunoglobulin.

**NATURE OF THE VACCINE.** Vaccines must be handled so that they do not lose their antigenicity. Live virus vaccines, in particular, seldom contain enough antigen to immunize an animal unless the virus can infect and replicate in the host. Inactivated vaccines have a large antigenic mass but, in general, must be administered several times to induce an adequate and protective immune response. At this time there are no absolute answers to the question of whether to use modified live or inactivated vaccines. In general, modified live viral vaccines are more efficacious and provide a longer period of immunity than inactivated vaccines, although there are exceptions. On occasion, live virus products raise safety questions on vaccine-induced diseases that are absent with inactivated vaccines, particularly when vaccines are administered to a species other than the one for which they are intended. However, both types of vaccines have their place in immunization programs. A related problem occurred in the Newcastle disease virus eradication program in California; vaccinated birds remained healthy following exposure but became infected and shed large quantities of virus. Thus, the vaccinates acted as potential sources for other birds and flocks (USDA 1978). Adjuvants may be added to killed products to help stimulate immunity, although some of the most effective adjuvants cannot be used in vaccines because of severe or undesirable side reactions.

**ROUTE OF VACCINATION.** Manufacturers' directions should be followed explicitly when administering vaccines, i.e., if an intramuscular route is recommended, the vaccine should not be given subcutaneously, or vice versa. Administering the vaccine by the wrong route may result in failure to produce immunity.

The question of parenteral versus local immunization requires a thorough understanding of the pathogenesis of the disease. Intranasal immunization has the advantage of inducing local antibody as well as local CMI in the respiratory tract. However, if the specific agent replicates systemically and not locally in the epithelial cells lining the respiratory tract, there will be no advantage to local over parenteral immunization. The virus of bovine virus diarrhea, frequently considered to be intestinal, is known to replicate initially in lymphoid tissue. An oral product offers no advantage in this situation. Similarly, feline panleukopenia is a disease frequently considered to be an enteric infection; however, the virus replicates first in the lymphoid tissue and later infects cells of the gastrointestinal tract. In this instance, not only is oral immunization less efficacious than parenteral immunization, but also it has been found to be without effect unless there is simultaneous intranasal immunization. An attempt should be made to protect the primary site of infection, therefore, local immunization may be more efficacious when the primary site of replication is the respiratory or gastrointestinal tract.

**AGE OF RECIPIENT.** Age is important not only because of the persistence of colostral antibody, but also because of the relative immunologic unresponsiveness that occurs during the neonatal period in many species. Although humoral immunity does not appear to be influenced to the same extent as CMI, antibody response would be affected.

There also is evidence suggesting that animals in the later years of life may have a decreased ability to produce antibody, as well as a decreased CMI response. Periodic revaccination during these later years, therefore, is particularly important to maintain an active state of immunity.

**NUTRITIONAL CONDITION.** A severely debilitated individual may not respond adequately to a vaccine, therefore, adequate nutritional levels should be maintained to insure that nutritional factors do not interfere with the immune response. To insure adequate protection when a debilitated animal is vaccinated, the vaccination should be repeated when the animal's general condition has improved. Also, caution should be exercised when using modified live viruses in a debilitated animal, since apparent attenuation of virulence is dependent on the host as well as the agent.

**CONCURRENT INFECTION.** It is important that subjects to be immunized are not already incubating the disease. Interest in vaccination rises when the risk of exposure increases. To prevent "vaccination breakdowns," prior to vaccination a detailed history should be taken concerning the possibility of exposure; a physical examination should be performed, if possible.

The presence of other diseases may result in immunosuppression, potentially interfering with the effectiveness of vaccination. For example, the general state of T-cell suppression present in hog cholera or bovine virus diarrhea may interfere with the response to vaccination or may contraindicate the use of live vaccines.

**DRUG TREATMENTS.** Vaccines should *not* be given concurrently with immunosuppressive drug treatment such as cyclophosphamide, azathioprine, methotrexate, and corticosteroids. Attenuated viruses should be harmless in a normal host but may produce clinical disease in an immunologically compromised host. High doses of steroids are known to reactivate bovine herpesvirus and possibly other herpesviruses (equine viral rhinotracheitis virus, pseudorabies). As such, they potentially could cause infection in susceptible contacts.

## Vaccines in Perspective

There is a tendency to rely on indiscriminate mass vaccination as a major tool in bringing diseases under control and eradicating pathogens. Although a good vaccine is a valuable tool, any tool can be misused; vaccines are no exception. The smallpox eradication program is an instance where early mass vaccination programs gave way to selectively applied vaccination efforts in order to increases effectiveness and efficiency.

In India in 1962, a mass vaccination program was begun; in 5 years, more than 500 million people were vaccinated. In 1967, when WHO began its push in India, smallpox was as prevalent as ever, in spite of the previous vaccination program. Some of the reasons for this were (1) the same people received multiple vaccinations (particularly school children), (2) the lower income groups were not reached in many cases, and (3) the vaccine was not stable enough to give adequate protection (CDC 1979c). Blind mass vaccination is often a waste of time, vaccine, and personnel. Mass vaccination campaigns should continue in endemic areas, but surveillance, investigation, and selective epidemiologic control techniques are of equal and, under certain circumstances, even greater importance than systematic mass vaccination (Foege et al. 1971).

Vaccines usually play a more important role in control programs than in final eradication efforts because some vaccines prevent disease but not infection, and others may produce lasting antibody response that interferes with diagnostic testing.

When different serovars or strains provide little or no cross-protection against each other, as in leptospirosis, foot-and-mouth disease, and influenza, major efforts are required to assure the vaccine used is proper and current.

Proper storage is necessary to maintain the effectiveness of vaccines, however, storage conditions are often less than optimum in the locale where the actual injections will be given: electric power sources may be sporadic or unavailable in many parts of the world, and even in industrialized countries, livestock in need of vaccine are likely to be hours away from the nearest electric outlet. Consequently, the cold-chain concept, maintaining a chain of refrigeration from production to inoculation, has developed. Although lyophilization has reduced the necessity for low temperatures for a few vaccines, an unbroken cold chain is an absolute necessity for most immunization programs.

Maintaining a cold chain demands detailed logistical planning and precise execution to meet the requirements of both the vaccine and the program. Items such as cold boxes, kerosene-powered refrigerators, and backup emergency generators are valuable assets; however, the irreplaceable factor is a conscientious, competent, and well-trained staff.

It is important that the public be informed of the limitations as well as the benefits of vaccination. Too often, vaccines are regarded as magic cure-alls that will provide total protection against disease merely by injecting every individual that can be persuaded, or restrained, to stand for it. This ignores the fact that vaccines, dramatic and valuable as they are, are but one tool. Disease prevention, control, and eradication programs do not succeed with vaccination alone, but vaccines can be a key element of a successful effort if the affected public is provided with a balanced understanding.

# 11

# Public Relations, Education, and Information

ALTHOUGH MANY ASPECTS of public relations, education, and information are intertwined, the differences in objectives are significant. Public relations, the only one of the three aimed totally at the public, is essentially a matter of creating a positive feeling toward a program or institution. Education, on the other hand, is the presentation of specific facts that the audience should know about a program. In disease control, these facts concern disease prevalence, costs, signs, transmission, program objectives and procedures, or similar items. The intent is to increase the level of understanding of the disease problem and solution. Information has more of a current news-release flavor and can be described as keeping the audience informed of the status and developments of a given program.

The broad program-oriented objectives of these subjects are fourfold: (1) to convert public apathy into useful action, (2) to gain the support of industry and society, (3) to agree on technical facts, and (4) to reconcile in understandable terms, the differences between local beliefs and the facts.

It is generally accepted that a change in attitude must precede a change in behavior (Cohen 1964). Human behavior plays a major role in the occurrence of disease, and the final purpose of education and information is not merely to present facts but to have them implemented; to induce permanent, positive, behavioral changes.

There are both technical and educational aspects of disease prevention, and it is important that the educational efforts begin as early as possible (Gordon 1963). Once controversy develops, people tend to choose sides first, then search for data that will support their contention (Ross 1973). Objective information is far more effective if presented before polarization occurs. It is important to remember that society, including the affected industry, initially may not view a disease problem in the same light as regulatory officials.

Unless a disease is recognized as significant by the affected industry, there will be little support for a solution. It is important to try to view a program through the eyes of the affected groups. By doing so, the program planners will not only be imparting information, but will be receiving it as well. Only by listening and keeping an open mind can we learn what is important, what is expected from a program, and what the citizens are prepared to accept. If those affected are not willing to accept what must be done, mutual exchange of ideas must continue until a consensus can be reached that does not compromise required program procedures.

## What Kind of Information?

Over the long range of a program the public should be kept informed of the progress of that program: are the short term goals being met, is the program on target in terms of time and space, what problems are being encountered, where, if necessary, is additional public support needed? There are times when feedback is as important as traceback. The affected industry also must be apprised of the need for maintaining vigil after the disease agent has been eradicated so that future introductions will be detected quickly, reported promptly, and dealt with adequately.

Policy decisions on public relations, education, and information must consider confidentiality when infections are discovered and quarantines imposed. What is the proper balance between an owner's right of confidentiality and the public's (including their adjacent neighbors) need to know for their own protection? Because they bear the public's trust, program officials not only have certain authority in terms of their informational emphasis, omissions, sequence of releases, and timing throughout the program, they also have comparable responsibilities in each area. During the U.S. hog cholera eradication program, a "minute-man" warning system was planned nationally but responsibility for administration was local. In addition to media notices stating that infection was in the area, personal visits were made to owners in a predefined radius around the infection, warning of the risk of exposure and leaving educational material on what precautions to take. Infected herds were not identified specifically; the neighborhood grapevine accomplished this without the benefit of the government. It is vital that deserved credit be given to cooperating agencies, industry members, practitioners, and other individuals in the community.

A balanced view of the program must be maintained. For example, in rabies control programs there is a tendency to focus on vaccination to the exclusion of stray dog control and bite investigations. Also, in the screwworm program most people think of a sterile fly distribution program and are unaware of the importance of surveillance and management practices such as wound treatment and timing of surgery and births. Although the public should be aware of the government's contribution to a program, it is even more important that people understand their own role. Industry and the general public cannot fulfill their part without such an understanding. They must accept the problem as their own and be actively involved in its solution.

Burridge and Schwabe (1977) emphasized the importance of the public knowledge in disease control programs; in echinococcosis programs, the dog owner is the unit of concern, not the dog, for the owner permits his dog to gain access to raw offal.

Public acceptance cannot be obtained unless the request that is made of them is consistent with their beliefs and standards (e.g., slaughter of infected cattle or destruction of stray dogs would not be tolerated in Hindu or Buddhist cultures).

Culture impinges on diseases and their control in many ways, including decisions on whether a given condition should even be considered as disease or as a natural state of life (Miller 1973). Although most health workers would accept that social and cultural beliefs influence the probability of exposure to agents, few would go so far as to consider that disease is a social and cultural phenomenon as well as a biological one. Beran and Gregorio (1966) pointed out that sociologic problems in disease control are far more difficult to solve than the technologic ones. If producers do not understand or believe in infectious agents and transmission chains, they are not likely to grant wholehearted support to programs based on these concepts. The educational aspect of the program must not only deal with the specifics of the problem, it must some times be aimed toward changing social and cultural beliefs. Whereas health professionals would view crowded human living quarters shared with sick animals as a serious health hazard, the owner may consider crowded conditions as normal and sharing them with sick animals an essential part of the cure, either as a means of improving nursing care or by placating displeased deities.

## Preparation and Presentation

Public relations, education, and information usually center around prepared releases distributed to mass media such as newspapers, magazines, radio, and television stations. Although of limited effectiveness on their own, as part of a total effort these releases can go far toward accomplishing program objectives if competently prepared and tailored to fit the needs of the program, the particular media, and the community in question. Be aware that while we remember only 10% of what we read, we remember 50% of what we hear and see. A well illustrated, properly presented oral presentation, with adequate audience participation is worth the investment of time required for preparation.

Every effort should be made to work with the media through every phase of a program, not just the kickoff formalities. However, it is unrealistic to expect every program release to be used. The acceptance will be much greater if the releases are concise, understandable and readable, have local appeal, and have been prepared by someone with reporting experience. In many situations where it seems probable that disease agents will be introduced into a community, it would be wise to prepare background information on the disease and circulate advance copies to the media. Then, when the problem arises, responsible writers will have readily available, factual, basic material on the disease and will not be forced to rely on secondhand information or misinformed sources. Each release should include a name and telephone number where additional information can be obtained.

Assuming the population characteristics are known, all materials should be tailored to the individual community in terms of its needs, abilities, beliefs, perceptions, language, and educational level. Ordinarily this tailoring requires professional help, such as a specially trained information specialist who can function as a two-way communicator, securing feedback information as well as distributing it.

All presentations should be simple, accurate, and interesting. They are valueless if they are not understood. If the various presentations are inconsistent or are open to widespread disbelief, they are doomed to failure. If presentations are not interesting, the subject matter will be ignored. As a professional, you may well accept a boring presentation merely because you feel a definite need to know, however, such a burning desire for knowledge will not be found in general audiences.

Individuals learn at various speeds and for various reasons; thus, in most programs there will be a small segment of the population that resists education by all methods of presentation. When all other forms of education have failed, and only after there has been enough preparation with the judicial branch to assure that the end result will be positive for the program, the last resort is enforcement with legal action and fines or other penalties. When self-benefit is not immediate and evident, or when the action is inconvenient and persuasion alone reaches only a small proportion of the population, the enforcement aspects must be well advertised. This is somewhat akin to using a stick when training a mule; the first step is to get the animal's attention. However, as stressed earlier, a blend of compulsion and good education is essential for success.

In many instances, word of mouth may be far more important to the long-term success of a program than official media. Often, the most effective method of gaining public acceptance is through acceptance and presentation by peers. One method of achieving this acceptance is the formation of local committees to assist in organizing and conducting the program, improving liaison with other industry members, increasing community understanding of the program, avoiding potential problems, dealing with difficult situations that arise locally, and exerting peer pressure on recalcitrants.

Chain (1979) outlined, in question form, a planning strategy for an informational program as follows:

1. Which communication channels (mass or interpersonal) are best suited for the motivational (awareness) phase?

2. Which motivational content is most effective for the target audience? Remember that the program administrators and clients may have different ideas of what is appealing.

3. What is the best medium for the informative phase?

4. What is the best informational content? Will the audience relate to the people, dress, and environment in the visual aids to facilitate proper interpretation of the message?

5. What is the best consultative channel? Can program officials establish and maintain a two-way dialogue, being good listeners as well? Are they receptive to field information? Are they flexible when community feedback suggests a change is needed? Do they effectively debrief field personnel periodically?

6. Is there a system for evaluating the communication program?

To answer these questions the communicator must not only understand the program but also have studied the target audience(s) to determine what is needed and how it should be presented.

## Role of Government

Ideally, citizens should claim a public program against disease as their own rather than a government idea thrust upon them, each person accepting personal responsibility for safeguarding the health of others, including his neighbors' animals. The importance of this philosophy was illustrated in the report of the National Brucellosis Technical Commission (1978a), which pointed out that in some states the burden of finding infected animals fell upon government agencies, with some segments of the cattle industry either taking no action for disease prevention or, in some cases, taking actions that increased spread of the pathogen. In other states, economic and accountability incentives influenced members of the industry to assume individual responsibility to protect their own and neighboring herds. The commission recommended that the USDA and the states revise the rules under which the program then operated to shift from sole government responsibility for locating disease to a shared responsibility, with a greater governmental emphasis on diagnosis and individual herd planning, and legal recourse against those who take actions that increase the spread of brucellosis.

It is important to realize that the personal and professional conduct of the program employees (from the lowest paid worker to the director), in terms of their knowledge, appearance, and attitude, does much to influence the eventual success of the program. As long as any viewer associates them with the program, their routine, casual, daily contacts with people play an important role in public relations. For example, what is your reaction when an automobile speeds recklessly past you on the highway and then pulls sharply in front you? If that automobile bears official markings, the image of the organization suffers. A program employee who is rude, discourteous, overbearing, or insensitive can do a great deal of damage. All employees should be competent, generally familiar with the overall program, and attentive to the problems of the public resulting from the program. If they are unable to resolve a citizen's problem personally, they should immediately and courteously refer the inquiry to a person who can provide the needed assistance, remembering the citizen usually is not there voluntarily but because of program demands or inconveniences. Remember, the employee is a member of a tax-supported agency that belongs to the public and exists only because the public wills it to do so.

## Role of the Community

Within a community, special emphasis should be given to the opinion makers, who may or may not be the official leaders of the community. Whether they hold public office or are wealthy, these persons are the pacesetters for the community; whatever they accept and do the community accepts and follows, for personal influence is a powerful force in creating behavioral change (Chaffee 1972). It is vital to the success of a program that these persons be identified and convinced before the program begins. Also, it is important to incorporate social, political, and religious leaders; churches; schools; and service clubs. If information is heard in a familiar, trusted situation from a person whose opinion is valued, the citizens will be far more receptive to the material presented.

Person to person communication is by far the most effective method of transmitting information. Frequently, this is the only way some individuals will be reached. In some situations, presentation at schools (including handouts and perhaps poster contests for the children), can be most effective, not only in obtaining immediate support for a particular program, but also in long-range formation of an educated public. In other situations the market place is a natural forum for informational and educational material. It is important to use as many methods of information dissemination as possible.

## Role of Industry

An effective method of reaching industry and professional groups is to maintain liaison with their associations and membership and maintain active participation with these groups if possible. This contact with others may yield even greater benefits to an open mind. Cattle producers believed ticks were important in Texas fever transmission long before scientists were willing to seriously consider such a possibility. One technique for furthering this liaison is the formation of advisory groups with strong industry representation.

People who recognize the problems and costs of a given disease are better able to understand the benefits of a successful control or eradication program. These benefits may include not only avoidance of continuing financial costs but also lessened psychological damage and loss of reputation. Industry should not, however, expect more from the program than the program is able to deliver. Exactly what results are anticipated and the expected time required to accomplish these results should be known. A control program should never be sold as an eradication effort, nor should the results be presented in an overly optimistic manner in an attempt to achieve immediate acceptance by industry. Acceptance will deteriorate rapidly and revert to antagonism if the program does not meet industry expectations.

It also is important that industry understands exactly what will be required in terms of operational changes, expenditures, and inconveniences related to the program, including when and where quarantines may be invoked, how and under what circumstances tests will be conducted, whether testing or vaccination will be required or optional, who is to pay for the procedures, what will be done when infected animals are disclosed, what marketing restrictions will be placed on herds, and whether or not indemnities will be available to assist the owner. Industry and society should be aware of what program they are "buying," why they are buying it, and the price, rather than being asked to sign a blank check.

## Role of the Health Professionals

There are important ethical and philosophical questions involved in all aspects of public relations, education, and information, since these carry with them all the implications of managed media. Career professionals may assume that their decisions are innately correct, that right is on their side, and there is a strong tendency in such a psychological environment to feel that such a meritorious objective as disease eradication justifies some information "management" to reach the goal. Health workers tend to become so obsessed with program objectives that they forget the concerns of the people they are dealing with. Occasional injections of the social sciences into the biological sciences will help keep this problem to a minimum and lead to programs that do things with people, not for or to them (Hanlon and Pickett 1979). Public information should be presented with the same objectivity required in approaching professional colleagues.

One of the immediate aims of an educational program must be to reach the scientific community and gain its support before approaching the public. Ideally, all members of that community will agree on the extent of the problem, the necessity for attacking it, and the means by which the problem can best be solved. This will not come about without a lengthy interchange of views and information with the health professionals and gradual development of a consensus regarding scientific facts on the disease. Such items as the route of transmission, reservoir, incubation period, clinical signs, diagnostic tests, prevalence, and treatment need to be presented uniformly to avoid confusing the public.

The mutual exchange of information also should include members of the legislative and executive branches of government, for the support of both is essential if the program is to be soundly conceived, financed, and enforced.

The difficulty in convincing health professionals of their importance in information and education was stressed by Gelfand (1973) when he suggested that the entire orientation of medical education was in need of marked changes. He also stated that there are important elements of persuasion in compulsory public health in a democratic society: the public and its elected representatives must be persuaded to pass laws requiring compulsion, and the public and those responsible for enforcement must be persuaded to accept the requirement for acts of individual compulsion. However, pure persuasion, including everything from simple appeals to true health education and understanding, generally produces far less effective programs.

# 12

## Applying Epidemiologic Principles

THE BASIC OBJECTIVE of the epidemiologic approach is to define the factors that interact to maintain a disease agent. Although the approaches for different diseases may vary markedly, the principles are the same. Most of the commonly encountered problems stem from our preoccupation with disease agents when the problem should be considered holistically. The concept of multiple causation should be utilized, realizing that disease does not result from the etiologic agent alone, but from a complex interaction of agent, host, and environment.

Eradication is the converse of agent maintenance (Yorke et al. 1979), therefore, only by recognizing and utilizing multiple causation as it results in agent perpetuation can control and eradication programs proceed efficiently. Since illness and infestation occur only in individuals that are both exposed and susceptible, we must uncover those factors that predispose to exposure and susceptibility.

A major objective is to break the web of transmission; thus, it immediately becomes apparent that the entire cycle of transmission must be considered rather than focusing on only one aspect. This cycle includes such factors as reservoirs, sources, portals of exit, potential routes of transmission (including vehicles and vectors), and portals of entry.

### Ecologic Factors

Agent factors to consider include pathogenicity, virulence, immunogenicity, immunogenic portion, antigenic stability, viability, size, incubation period, host range and physical factors, and environment.

Pathogenicity, the ability to produce disease, and virulence, the severity of disease produced, influence control and eradication in two major ways. Highly pathogenic or virulent agents, because of the frequency or dramatic nature of the disease produced, are most liable to be the target of control or eradication efforts. As such agents are relatively more visible, these factors also facilitate identification of cases after the program has started.

Immunogenicity is the ability of an agent to stimulate immunity in a host; e.g., hog cholera and African swine fever (ASF) have similar clinical pictures, but the viruses vary markedly in immunogenicity. Hog cholera virus is highly immunogenic and rapidly stimulates effective antibody production in the host, a characteristic that enables the development of vaccines that produce a long-lasting immunity. On the other hand, infection with ASF virus is characterized by a lack of production of neutralizing antibodies usually associated with humoral protection. This suggests that it will be difficult to develop a satisfactory vaccine against ASF virus.

Immunogenic portion refers to the mode of action of protective antibody, whether the antibody is formed in response to the agent itself or to one of its products. For example, protective antibodies are formed against the rabies virus, therefore, immunization prevents infection. However, protective antibody is formed against the tetanus toxin rather than against the organism, therefore, tetanus immunization prevents disease but does not prevent an animal from harboring the organism. The implications for control or eradication programs are obvious.

Antigenic stability refers to the probability that the genome governing the antigenic structure of an agent will undergo antigenic changes, i.e., mutation. Influenza virus strains affecting humans are notoriously unstable, mutating or recombining frequently, which results in a steady supply of susceptible hosts and almost an annual obsolescence of vaccines. This problem also developed in the United States when virulent hog cholera virus and hyperimmune serum were used simultaneously for immunizing swine. In 1949 a variant virus appeared in some of the commercial virus, thus, hyperimmune serum prepared from, and tested against, a standard hog cholera virus strain failed to protect against the undetected mutant when used in the recommended dosage. As a result field outbreaks of hog cholera occurred in swine that had received simultaneous injections of hyperimmune serum and the variant virus (USDA 1962). Canine distemper, on the other hand, has remained highly stable antigenically, with one vaccine protecting against strains that possess markedly different virulence.

Another aspect of genetic instability of microbial agents is the development of antibiotic resistance, as seen in the enterobacters. Genetic instability does, however, have a positive aspect: it is used to our advantage when organisms are manipulated in laboratories in attempts to produce strains with high immunogenicity yet low virulence and pathogenicity.

The viability of an organism, its ability to withstand environmental stresses, is extremely important in control efforts. Environmental decontamination is much simpler and more effective when dealing with the leptospires than with the agent of scrapie merely because of the difference in viability of the infectious agents. Leptospires are extremely fragile, being killed by mild acids or drying, whereas the scrapie agent can even withstand boiling.

Probably the most important control-related aspect of agent size is the effect it has on ease of transmission. For example, the ease with which an agent penetrates the respiratory tree is dependent to a great degree on the size of the pathogen (Bers 1973).

There are both control advantages and disadvantages when an agent has a short incubation period; e.g., surveillance of individuals known to have been exposed to foot-and-mouth disease (FMD) virus can be limited to a short time, but reporting and traceback must be rapid to interrupt transmission. Conversely, a long incubation period (e.g., scrapie), allows a more leisurely approach.

The importance of host range is that the greater the number of host species in which a disease agent can survive, the greater the probability is that it will survive, as illustrated by the salmonellae. As a general rule agents with a narrow host range, such as hog cholera virus, are more susceptible to control and eradication.

The physical factors of the host that are important as disease determinants include pathogenic state, nutritional state, physiological adaptation, sex, age, species, genetic makeup, and occupation or use to which the host is put. Many of these factors can be utilized by health agencies to make the most efficient use of their resources by determining high-risk individuals or groups.

Some of these factors, such as age and pathogenic state, are dynamic factors within individuals. Others, such as nutritional state, are dynamic on the herd level. Increasing reproductive rates or dramatically prolonging reproductive life alters the age structure of the herd. Another manifestation of the importance of age is the reduced incidence of an agent when calves are segregated from adults in herds infected with bovine leukosis (Wilesmith and Lorenz 1979) or tuberculosis (Dept. of Primary Industry 1979).

Environment, the last category of ecologic factors, may exert an effect on the agent, vehicle, vector, reservoir, or host. The factors to consider are virtually limitless but include such items as weather, housing, geography, geology, management practices, noise, air quality, and chemicals. Although few of these can be manipulated by health agencies, an understanding of their association with disease occurrence is vital to planning an efficient program. The importance of weather in restricting the spread of virus is illustrated in the first three outbreaks of FMD in the United States. All three outbreaks died out with little human assistance because heavy winter snows immobilized cattle and, to a large extent, even their human attendants (Hagan 1958).

Not all weather influences are so positive, however. During a smallpox program in Bangladesh in 1974, there was great optimism when only 91 infected villages were located. Unfortunately, most of these villages were in an area ravaged first by floods, then by famine, resulting in a massive dispersion of refugees, which was a major factor in the explosion of cases that peaked with 1208 infected villages by late April, 1975 (Henderson 1976).

## Transmission Cycles

**RESERVOIR.** Transmission occurs as a cycle, and discussion can begin at any segment; however, the most logical point is the natural habitat of the agent, the reservoir. Regardless of whether the reservoir is in animals or in some inanimate location such as soil, the magnitude of a reservoir is a major determinant of the probability of exposure to the agent. Eradication is vastly more difficult without knowledge of the reservoir.

Appearances can be misleading, for in many diseases the reservoir is not obvious. Most clinical cases of Eastern equine encephalitis occur in horses, humans, and pen-raised pheasants, whereas wild bird species constitute the reservoir.

It is important to differentiate between source and reservoir: the reservoir is where the agent resides, and the source is the place, object, or individual from which the agent passes immediately to a new host. The source may be a vehicle, vector, reservoir, or another host. To illustrate, in Venezuelan equine encephalitis, the source is a mosquito, but the significant reservoir is Equidae.

Animate reservoirs also may be termed maintenance hosts, characterized by becoming infected with regularity and shedding over a long time (Audy 1958). Other factors common to maintenance hosts are their high susceptibility, low clinical response, long-term shedding, and natural transmission within the species. Incidental hosts may be highly susceptible but do not shed large numbers of pathogens over a long time.

Geographic sites that persist as reservoirs for an extended time are referred to as nidi or nests (Audy 1958; Pavlovsky 1966). Of necessity, a nidus will be associated with a biotype that supports the reservoir and any essential vectors. The tenacity of a nidus depends to a large degree on the difference between the maintenance requirements of the reservoir and the amount of these elements in the biotype. Eradication probably will progress more rapidly in those areas with the thinnest maintenance margin, for the agent will lead a more tenuous existence there.

**PORTAL OF EXIT.** Obviously, to spread, an infectious agent must escape from the reservoir with sufficient frequency and in large enough numbers to constitute a source of infection for other hosts. The route by which the agent escapes is termed the portal of exit. For example, in bovine brucellosis, the most important portals of exit are uterine contents and milk. If no susceptible host contacts these substances, an event susceptible to management practices, the transmission cycle is broken. The importance of uterine contents in bovine brucellosis is shown in the statement by Hugh-Jones et al. (1976) that the time required to eliminate *Brucella abortus* from a herd is influenced more by the pregnancy status of the infected cows (thus their importance as potential sources) than by the number of infected cows.

The relative importance of the host in transmission of disease agents often is related to the portal of exit. Dogs and sheep constitute the definitive and intermediate hosts, respectively, for *Echinococcus granulosus*. Dogs shed the agent in their feces and can infect many sheep quickly. Conversely, sheep must be eaten uncooked for transmission to occur, so many never infect another host.

**ROUTE OF TRANSMISSION.** Having established the portal of exit, the next consideration is the route of transmission, how the agent travels from host to host. Transmission can occur either horizontally, between contemporaries, or vertically, from the parent (usually the mother) to the offspring, before or during birth or through the mother's milk. Emphasis here will be on horizontal transmission although vertical transmission can be important in maintaining agents that usually are transmitted horizontally (Plommet et al. 1971).

Horizontal transmission is either direct or indirect, with the distinction being the absence or presence of an intermediary. Direct transmission occurs via contact, injection, inhalation, or ingestion; indirect transmission involves either a vehicle or vector as an intermediary. Diseases transmitted by contact include venereal diseases or even such noninfectious events as insecticide poisonings. Infectious agents transmitted by injection include rabies, where a tooth is the inoculating weapon, or hookworm, where the agent itself is capable of burrowing through healthy skin. The act of coughing or sneezing produces airborne droplets of many sizes; larger droplets are projected a few feet and fall quickly to the ground. When another individual is infected by these droplets before they settle, it is termed direct droplet transmission. Some smaller droplets have such a low-moisture content that the water evaporates almost as soon as the droplet is expelled. These evaporated particles, termed droplet nuclei, may remain suspended in the air for an indefinite time and be carried over long distances. In this situation, air becomes a vehicle and transmission is indirect rather than direct.

By definition, indirect transmission involves either a vehicle or a vector and requires that the agent be capable of survival outside the host. The difference between a vehicle and a vector is that a vehicle is an inanimate object such as air, water, milk, other foods, or soil; a vector is a living animal or plant.

Vectors also can be subdivided, the usual division being mechanical versus biological. A mechanical vector is a vector in which the agent does not undergo any essential change during its association, whether the agent is carried internally or externally. Within a biological vector, agent changes might be simple multiplication, as occurs with plague bacilli in infected fleas; maturation of the agent, such as *Dirofilaria immitis* in mosquitoes; or sexual reproduction, as with malaria parasites in mosquitoes. In many instances, the agents are transmitted vertically in arthropod vector species via transovarial (from parent to young via ova) or transstadial (through nymphal stages to adult) passage.

Frequently, vectors such as mosquitoes and flies facilitate geographic spread of infectious agents by providing a degree of mobility that is not otherwise available. However, agent mobility is limited when the vector has a restricted host preference, as is the case with cattle tick fever or when the preferential host has a restricted home range. Although it is possible to find a suitable vector without finding the agent, the agent cannot persist in an area that is not inhabited by its required vector.

**PORTAL OF ENTRY.** Having progressed from the reservoir through the portal of exit and route of transmission, the next consideration is the portal of entry, the means by which an agent enters a new host. Often portals of entry and exit are in the same system, for example, the respiratory tract for influenza and the gastrointestinal tract for salmonellae. However, this generalization is far from constant. Similarly, the portal of entry frequently is suggested by the clinical picture, as in Newcastle disease where the signs suggest a respiratory portal, or in footrot where the portal is the skin of the foot.

It is not unusual for an agent to utilize multiple portals of entry, possibly with serious control implications. Entry of *Coxiella burnetii* (agent for Q fever) through the intestinal tract in milk can be controlled quite simply by pasteurization. However, when the portal of entry is the respiratory tract, control is much more difficult.

**CYCLE INTERRUPTION.** The time required to complete the entire cycle of transmission varies with each agent, but it is an observable epidemiologic unit referred to as the serial interval. It reflects, to some extent, the life cycle of the parasite and influences the frequency of testing and treatment necessary in control programs.

Agents with complex life cycles are more amenable to eradication than those with simple life cycles; i.e., complex life cycles present greater opportunities for effective intervention because the agent has multiple requirements that must be met for its continued survival. Eradication of cattle tick fever from the United States was not accomplished by attacking the pathogen (*Babesia bigemina*) but by eliminating its obligate intermediate host tick.

The classification of diseases used by Schwabe (1969) is helpful since it offers valuable insight into organization of eradication programs. He described five categories based on life cycles: direct, cyclo, meta, sapro, and special.

Direct diseases, such as brucellosis and foot-and-mouth disease, require only one vertebrate host for their cycle, which is relatively simple and may be difficult to disrupt.

The cyclozoonoses, most of which are cestode infections, require two vertebrate species to complete their cycle. An example is *Taenia saginata,* which requires both cattle and humans for its perpetuation, thus presenting greater opportunities for breaking the cycle.

Metazoonoses, such as the arboviruses, must have both a vertebrate and an invertebrate host for survival, raising the possibility of attacking the vector rather than the definitive host.

Ancylostomiasis is one of the saprozoonoses, depending on both a verte-brate host and a nonanimal source, in this instance, soil. Environmental ma-nipulation can be an effective control for agents with this type of cycle.

The special zoonoses, such as *Erysipelothrix* infections and tularemia, can be maintained by more than one cycle. Although one cycle may be susceptible to intervention, the alternative cycle may foil eradication efforts.

Communicable diseases most commonly spread through a population at a geometric rather than an arithmetic rate. This spread is expressed as an infec-tion potential and is measured as the secondary case rate that varies by disease, route of transmission, and level of herd immunity. The rate of spread also is determined by such things as the number of sources and agent infectivity. Surprisingly, even with highly infectious agents this rate of spread is manage-able. For example, persons infected with smallpox were found to spread the agent to only two or three other persons on the average and most of this transmission occurred with the infected household (Foege et al. 1971).

### Infectivity

Merely entering the body of a new host is not sufficient to produce infection; the agent also must multiply and produce a change. However, this change is not necessarily harmful to the host, for it could be limited to something as benign as a serologic response or a biochemical alteration. The epidemiologi-cally important occurrences in the infectious process begin with exposure, for unless the agent invades the host in sufficient numbers to produce infection, the exposure is of no consequence.

When there is exposure to the agent in sufficient numbers to be infective for a new host, communicability becomes a concern. The mean interval be-tween exposure and beginning of communicability is referred to as the genera-tion period. This valuable information defines the rapidity of transmission and the speed with which an epidemic will build. Decreasing the rate of transmis-sion will produce a noticeable effect far more quickly in diseases with short generation periods, something to consider in program evaluation and public information. Depending on the agent, this period of communicability may be prior to, during, or after clinical disease.

In most infections, the host becomes free of the agent following recovery. In others, such as herpesvirus infections, the organism remains latent in the host and may be undetectable with usual laboratory techniques, yet reappears during times of stress. Another variation is with infections such as psittacosis and salmonellosis where the organism may be present in detectable amounts in the host but is shed only at intervals. In these situations, as in true latency, periods of shedding often are stress induced.

One of the most important deterrents to disease control is a carrier, an individual with a subclinical infection that is shedding the agent in infectious doses; i.e., the host is completely mobile and appears normal clinically, yet it has the ability to transmit the agent to other hosts or vectors. This condition occurs in the vast majority of infections known to medical science. Carriers may occur as incubationary, convalescent, intermittent, chronic, and healthy.

Incubationary carriers shed the agent in amounts sufficient to infect another host before they become ill themselves. For example, in FMD, cattle may shed the virus from the pharynx for 5 days prior to the onset of illness. This type of carrier presents obvious problems in control programs based on isolation of cases.

Convalescent carriers shed infectious amounts for a relatively short time after recovery from the illness, e.g., in feline leukopenia the infectious agent is shed in the urine or feces for only 3–6 weeks after recovery.

Intermittent carriers, as in typhoid fever, also shed during and after convalescence, but organisms are shed intermittently rather than continuously.

Tuberculosis, which often produces life-time shedders, illustrates the chronic state with shedding for months, years, or even life.

Probably the most dangerous from the standpoint of disease transmission are healthy carriers, which shed the agent but are never recognized as being clinically ill. For example, *Salmonella typhimurium* infections in normal swine can persist at least 6 months with intermittent shedding following stress situations over the entire period. The mobility and apparent good health of these animals make them much more efficient transmitters than animals that are recognized as sick and isolated from susceptible individuals.

While individual host resistance often determines whether that individual will have a subclinical infection or experience clinical disease, the exposing dose is also important. As a general rule, a large exposing dose will result in a shorter incubation period and more severe illness than a mild dose, especially with parasitic infections such as trichinosis, where the agent undergoes only one reproductive cycle in the definitive host. Any efforts that reduce the exposing dose can have a significant impact on the success of control programs.

The spectrum of infection varies from total health through inapparent infections; from mild, moderate, and severe clinical illness, to death. For example, in an outbreak of arboviral encephalitis in humans, 60% of those exposed might remain uninfected, 15% could develop antibodies while remaining healthy, 8% could have a mild, probably undiagnosed illness, 6% could experience moderate illness, 4% could suffer severe illness, and another 7% could die. The spectrum of infection varies according to the agent factors of infectivity, pathogenicity, and virulence, as well as individual host resistance and environmental stresses.

## Herd Immunity

Herd immunity is an epidemiologic concept that is not fully understood but one that plays an important role in disease control. It exists when the proportion of immune individuals becomes so great in a given population that, under ordinary circumstances, a communicable agent cannot be maintained. Immunity may be acquired either naturally or artificially, but if herd immunity is dependent on natural infection, the agent must be encountered with sufficient frequency to insure that a large proportion of individuals in the population is exposed and becomes immune. Under any circumstances, the immunity of each individual within the herd must be durable, effective, and must prevent transmission rather than just prevent disease.

The duration of herd immunity is influenced by such factors as the duration of immunity in each individual animal, addition of susceptible animals to the herd, departure of immunes through death and emigration, infectivity of the agent, ease of agent transmission, duration of shedding by infected animals, and interaction or degree of movement within the population. These general comments on herd immunity are made with the assumption that herd size and number of contacts remain constant and that contacts between susceptible animals and shedders within the herd are random.

Herd immunity operates by reducing the probability that susceptible animals will contact a transmitter. As the proportion of randomly distributed immune animals increases in a population, the proportion of susceptible animals in the immediate environment of a transmitting individual decreases. Therefore, the probability of successful transfer of an infectious agent decreases as the proportion of susceptible animals decreases. Increasing the number of immune individuals decreases the probability of an epidemic occurring only when it reduces the number of contacts between susceptibles and shedders. A key factor is the susceptible animal rather than the immune one, but the most critical factor is the frequency of contact among susceptible animals. An increase in these contacts (i.e., when the animals are gathered for vaccination) increases the epidemic potential. Similarly, if the number of susceptible contacts remains constant, the epidemic potential will remain constant despite the addition of an infinite number of immune animals to the herd.

Susceptible animals are added to a population through birth, immigration, or waning of individual immunity. A low rate of addition to a population results in well-separated waves of illness with intervening quiet periods. A high rate of addition, however, results in a high, relatively steady infection rate. The rate of population turnover varies markedly among species, being quite rapid in poultry and swine but very slow in humans. The contact rate among susceptible animals that is critical to maintain an agent in a given situation is determined by such factors as agent infectivity, stress, route of transmission, vector abundance, population density, and individual mobility. Highly infective agents such as the FMD virus are transmitted easily and can persist in a population with a relatively low contact rate between susceptibles and shedders. Agents with low infectivity, such as *Mycobacterium bovis,* require a much higher contact rate.

The critical contact rate is so vital to the maintenance of pathogens that chance culling is adequate to eradicate brucellosis from some herds (Hugh-Jones et al. 1976). Also, eradication of an agent will soon result in a highly susceptible population, which makes it essential that barriers be established that will prevent reintroduction of the agent.

Stress factors act essentially by reducing host resistance, thus increasing the ease of infection and reducing the dose required to produce infection. Similarly, an agent that can be transmitted by droplet nuclei can be maintained with a lower contact rate than an agent such as rabies virus that depends on bite transmission. Although an abundance of infective vectors facilitates transmission of vector-transmitted agents, the only situation in which acquired herd immunity is effective in eliminating vector-transmitted agents is when the host is also the reservoir.

Both dense populations and highly mobile individuals predispose to a high rate of contact among individuals, thereby increasing the probability of an epidemic. In large (not necessarily dense) populations that have a low contact rate, diseases with a long duration of immunity are most likely to be endemic, with long cycles and large fluctuations in incidence.

Acquired herd immunity is relative just as individual immunity is relative: as the proportion of susceptible individuals decreases in a population, the probability of direct transmission of a given infectious agent decreases also. As a result, epidemics of a specific disease become essentially impossible in a herd long before the proportion of immune individuals in the population reaches 100%. In small populations, herd immunity may cause infectious agents to disappear completely unless additional susceptible animals are introduced.

Conversely, in herds above a certain critical size, herd immunity may cause infections to remain at low levels until the new susceptible animals accumulate in numbers sufficient to permit a fresh outbreak. This critical number of susceptible animals needed to maintain endemicity within a herd is termed the "endemic threshold." Bartlett (1960) found that in urban areas, a population of less than 500,000 was not adequate to maintain measles endemicity. Anderson et al. (1981) pointed out that cycles of rabies are most common where fox densities are highest and frequently are absent in low-density populations. The interaction of hosts, contacts, and agents is a delicate balance, however, for it is quite likely that in two populations of the same size but of dissimilar density, a disease will burn itself out in the dense herd but will become endemic in the less dense one. The operative factor would be the difference in the secondary case rates, with the high rate in the dense herd rapidly exhausting the susceptible animals.

In interherd transmission, spread does not cease as a result of susceptible depletion; it decreases because dissemination becomes less favorable (Miller 1976). The dissemination rate is the number of new herds infected by each infected herd. This is the interherd counterpart of the secondary case rate.

Yorke et al. (1979) list seven factors that influence virus perpetuation: population size, turnover, density, and immunity; transmissibility; duration of infectiousness; and generation. This concept further states that introducing a transmitting individual into a community will not give rise to an outbreak if the density of susceptible animals is below another critical level, the "outbreak threshold." Once the outbreak threshold is exceeded, the outbreak will be of sufficient size to reduce the density of susceptible animals as far below the threshold as it originally was above the threshold, i.e., if the threshold is barely exceeded, the outbreak will be small but if the density of susceptible animals is far above the threshold, few susceptibles will remain when the outbreak has subsided.

When dealing with communicable diseases, herd immunity is applicable to a small family farm, a community, or even a national herd; however, random distribution is frequently ignored or overlooked. While a large herd might have 65% immunity, it is conceivable that it could be divided into two subgroups with considerable interaction within each, but no contact between the two. Furthermore, it is possible that one group could have 100% immunes and the other group 30% immunes; in such a situation a 65% immune figure is meaningless—herd immunity will not be operable. If immunization is to play a role in control efforts in a situation such as this, it is imperative that we overlook the 65% figure and concentrate instead on the two subgroup figures, 100% and 30%. Obviously, immunization programs should focus on the group at highest risk.

# 13

# Identifying Risk

HIGH-RISK GROUPS are those segments of a population with the greatest probability of experiencing a certain event. In our field of interest this event usually is a disease. For most efficient use of resources, prevention and control efforts should focus on the high-risk portion of the population.

The first prerequisite for determining a high-risk group is an accurate, effective surveillance program that gathers comprehensive information on the occurrence of disease. Analysis of accumulated data from individual epidemiologic studies will identify sources of outbreaks and define high-risk points, which assist in evaluation throughout the program, for risk factors change in relative importance as initial high-risk factors are reduced by program actions.

Geographic distribution must be studied as a part of risk determination. The pertinent factor is whether the area meets the needs of the pathogen; the agent can flourish where these requirements are fulfilled. Unless natural barriers exist (isolation, temperature, altitude, moisture), an agent will spread to contiguous areas that also meet its needs. Baltazard (1960) categorized ecologic areas as receptive (favoring pathogen entry and spread), critical (characterized as permanent foci), and immune (where the agent cannot enter or spread). Eradication efforts should center on critical areas and preventive measures should be taken to protect receptive areas; immune areas can be ignored.

Endemic and epidemic are two terms relative to disease distribution. Endemic is place oriented and refers to a geographic locality where a reasonably predictable number of cases occurs annually. Endemicity occurs when all factors have reached a balance in the population, assuring survival of both the agent and the host. Epidemic is time oriented and is a time of increased incidence. An epidemic can occur whenever there is an imbalance in favor of factors favoring the agent.

An essential item in determining whether an agent occurs in a given area is the suitability of that particular microenvironment. On grasslands, temperature may vary by as much as 11°C and humidity by as much as 20% between the ground surface and 1 meter above it. Many measurements are taken at places of convenience to humans, thus may not evaluate the suitability of the environment for the agent. It is important to put ourselves in the agent's place. To illustrate this concept in the malaria eradication program in India, Hinman (1966) stated that it was unnecessary to spray ceilings over 3 meters high since the primary vector did not rest above that level.

Recent events often play a major role in determining high-risk groups: a common food source in a food poisoning outbreak, hemorrhagic septicemia in newly introduced feeder cattle, distemper occurring after a dog show.

Another concept inherent in the study of high-risk groups is exposure potential, the probability that an individual will be exposed to a given disease agent. Any host factor may influence exposure potential. An obvious difference in exposure exists between open and closed populations; the increased freedom of movement in an open population means greater probability of exposure to most disease agents. Population movements such as occur in nomadism, pilgrimages, fairs, markets, seasonal agricultural pursuits, floods, famines, etc., are prime problems in disease control and eradication. Wilesmith and Lorenz (1979) reported that 89% of the bovine leukosis–infectd herds investigated in West Germany had been infected by purchasing infected cattle.

The exposure potential of herds also is related closely to the accumulation/liquidation cycle on farms. As cattle are added to a herd from various sources, the probability of exposure to pathogens rises dramatically. Conversely, during liquidation transmission is low for most animals are moving to slaughter, resulting in less interherd exchange of disease agents. This is the time to accelerate control and eradication efforts.

Age is extremely important in determining exposure potential. In most free-ranging species the very young are sheltered from other members of society except the immediate family and have very low resistance to most infectious diseases. As they mature, their mobility increases, increasing the probability of contact with other individuals and, therefore, disease agents. With old age, however, mobility decreases and reduces the exposure potential.

Rabies and canine distemper in owned dogs are diseases that illustrate this influence of age on susceptibility and exposure potential. Newborn pups are essentially 100% susceptible to rabies, but exposure is unlikely unless an exposing animal enters the nest. As the pups mature and mobility increases, the exposure potential increases, stabilizes, then gradually decreases as the dogs slow down with advanced age. Though the exposure potential increases, the susceptibility tends to decrease due to artificial immunization. With advanced age, the susceptibility may increase due to decreased immunization. However, it is possible that the importance of this decreased vaccination in older dogs is lessened by the long duration of immunity with present-day vaccines, especially in animals that have been vaccinated repeatedly.

The same approach to canine distemper produces an entirely different set of curves. Colostral antibodies protect most newborn pups, and only a small percentage are susceptible within a few hours after birth. This natural antibody degrades at a predictable half-life, thus increasing the number of susceptible animals; the percentage of susceptibles is lowered by passive and active immunization. Artificial intervention, coupled with long-lasting immunity from natural infection, results in a fairly rapid decrease of susceptibles during the first year or so of life, followed by a slowly declining percentage in later life.

One important but frequently overlooked fact in program evaluation is that the number of infections is much less informative than the percentage of the population affected (attack rate). Attack rates may be either crude or specific. The general formula is the number of occurrences (numerator) divided by the number of individuals at risk (denominator). The two parts must be consonant; e.g., in calculating a birthrate, only females of reproductive age are at risk, therefore only these females are included in the denominator.

Most rates are crude but they can and should be made specific by age, group, sex, or any other factor when the data are available. This specificity markedly improves comparability of different sets of data. A major problem encountered in calculating attack rates in veterinary medicine is the lack of denominator data anywhere but in selected herds. The data needed may be merely a population count by species or may include such factors as herd size, age, breed, sex, or management factors, depending on the problem. The characteristics of animal populations are difficult to gather but are important because of the variability among populations. For example, in one Illinois county only 15.6% of the dairy cattle were in herds of 11 or more animals, while 63.3% of the beef cattle were in such herds (Schnurrenberger et al. 1965).

Data on animal populations are scarce, and it is sometimes tempting to use those which are available, regardless of the source. For example, using herd brucellosis blood test charts as a source of accurate age data would be questionable, for young calves are not included and the ages of individuals tested are frequently noted in casual fashion. Also, cultural bias or superstition can be factors when field data are collected. In an outbreak of Western equine encephalitis, individual ages recorded for more than 200 horses investigated showed ages from less than 1 year to over 23 years, but not a single animal was recorded as having an age of 13 years (Doby et al. 1966).

From a broader standpoint, when experience has proven which indicators to look for in a particular disease, generally available information can be used in risk appraisal. In an endemic area a change in the prevalence of the risk indicators will be followed by an altered disease incidence. A common example of this relationship is the use of rainfall as a predictor of mosquito-borne viral encephalitis.

# 14

# Traceback
# and Identification

A CLASSIC DOCUMENTED EXAMPLE of an early outbreak investigation was John Snow's work during a 1680 cholera outbreak in London. His epidemiologic study traced back the source of the outbreak to a pump in Broad Street and was done long before bacteria were recognized as pathogens.

Today, proper traceback is a procedure that begins with a known infected individual, herd, or flock and traces all possible locational and interactive exposures in both directions, back toward the source and forward to contacts.

Moving backward toward the source begins with the date of onset of disease and conducts a retrospective examination of all movements of the individual during the maximum expected incubation period. When the date of onset and incubation period of a disease are relatively easy to determine, such as with foot-and-mouth disease or acute hog cholera, it is relatively easy to decide on the time period over which movement and contacts should be traced. However, with less evident diseases such as brucellosis, tuberculosis, or the chronic forms of hog cholera, subclinical infections are common and the onset is often insidious or obscure. In such cases, careful interview of the owner with attention to such factors as the mode of transmission, amount of infection in the herd, location of the infected animals within the herd, and intraherd movements will provide clues relative to how long the agent has been present. For example, with bovine brucellosis the most important portal of exit is the genital tract at the time of calving or abortion; therefore, it can be assumed that most intraherd transmission will occur at these times. A low level of infection suggests that the agent was introduced relatively recently. When infection is in only certain groups within the herd, reconstruction of intraherd movements may disclose, within fairly restrictive time limits, when the agent first entered the herd.

Obviously, animal identification procedures, detail and extent of the owner's records, owner's memory and cooperation, and investigative skills of the person performing the traceback all contribute to the success or failure of the traceback operation, not only in this phase, but in all others as well. It is vital to secure the trust and cooperation of the owner. Personal rapport may also help in situations where a farmer is reluctant to inform on his neighbors, fears law suits from persons who may have purchased infected livestock from him, or merely mistrusts government agencies.

After the proper time period for the investigation has been determined, it is essential to decide what type of information is needed. Again, knowledge of the important routes of transmission provides an answer. Is the agent spread by direct contact with carrier animals, water, feed, fomites, or arthropods? What is the reservoir? Answers to these questions will be a guide in deciding what further questions need to be asked. Do we need to know about livestock purchases, visits to sale barns or shows, livestock loans, farm visitors (including salesmen), broken fences, feed sources, wildlife harborage, or vector breeding sites? In addition to these specific questions, as much information as possible should be gathered about exposure incidents, including animal identification and description, date and location, and the name and address of each animal owner involved.

Retrospective traceback usually begins with the immediate neighbors of the index herd, but the investigation may finally span a continent. The search should not be terminated when the first possible source has been disclosed but should continue until all reasonable leads have been explored. Other cycles of infection that may be disclosed are just as important as the one involving the index herd.

When a probable source has been discovered, the search widens, for the agent did not originate at this location, it is merely one link in the chain of transmission. The source herd not only contracted the agent somewhere else, it could well have spread it to others in addition to the index herd. Rapid disclosure of these other potential new foci will abort additional outbreaks. The chain is more like a web, and every lead must be followed until no further progress can be made; either the trail becomes too cold for further pursuit or no further leads can be developed.

Concurrent with this retrospective study, a prospective investigation must be conducted to break the chain at the index point by promptly locating and placing under active surveillance all animals potentially infected by the index herd.

When dealing with movements with untraceable identification, an investigator must resort to more time-consuming means, such as charting all the marketing-point transactions and sorting out shippers and buyers, using records such as checks from buyers to sellers. False leads must be expected. The final case of hog cholera in Texas was found at a market and required locating and investigating 198 potential source herds in Texas and New Mexico before finding the one probable source. In addition, 88 receiving herds in Texas, New

Mexico, and Oklahoma were investigated with 30 being depopulated as potentially exposed (USDA 1981).

The costs of traceback when animal identification is missing are such that an obvious efficiency would result if marketed animals were routinely identified for future traceback should it be necessary. To be efficient, traceback markers involving abattoirs should be inexpensive, easy to apply, not invoke buyer resistance, be easily located and interpreted at the abattoir, and not interfere with slaughter (Watt 1979).

One example of an abattoir traceback is a cattle disease prevalence or monitoring program in the United States: the Market Cattle Identification (MCI) program, discussed in Chapter 7. In some Scandinavian countries where swine and other livestock are shipped directly to slaughter, the owner marks each animal so back-tracing to the farm is simple and rapid (Henricson 1975). The owner also is paid, in part, according to the health status of animals he sends to slaughter. This inducement improves cooperation in disease control programs.

The ease and efficiency of traceback vary with the complexity of the marketing system. In Queensland, Australia, where there are many large stations that sell directly to abattoirs without using intermediaries, traceback is a simple procedure using coded tail bands similar in concept to the MCI back tags; traceback is nearly 100% effective. In other regions, such as the United States, which have a more complicated market chain, back-tracing is much more difficult.

Konyha (1978) illustrated the cost-effectiveness of traceback procedures with the fiscal year 1977 data on bovine tuberculosis. One reactor animal was found for each 2175 cattle tested in trace-back investigations compared with one reactor for each 2,346,380 cattle tested in other programs. As a further example, traceback of one animal found to have suspicious lesions at slaughter resulted in disclosure of seven infected herds.

Traceback serves valuable functions other than case-finding. The investigations and interviews can provide insight into the management factors that promote and inhibit pathogen introduction into, and diffusion through, herds. Also, a functional system can provide a mechanism for monitoring the progress of a control program (Burridge and Schwabe 1977).

From the standpoint of disease control and eradication, it is evident that rapid traceback will produce more benefit, due to a rapid identification of sources, than a leisurely approach that permits a longer period of spread from such sources while they are being located. Speed is more important in infections with a short generation time. In an emergency program against a newly introduced disease capable of rapid spread, such as African swine fever or foot-and-mouth disease, immediate and exhaustive traceback is the key to preventing the establishment of the disease. Success in such situations requires the mobilization of enough personnel to follow each lead without delay, which requires many people in the field simultaneously, and also requires a well-organized command-post operation to assemble and analyze data and direct the investigators.

Four steps predicated upon identification are essential for a timely and ongoing traceback and surveillance system for livestock populations: (1) application of identification devices, (2) maintenance of herd-of-origin records, (3) recovery of the identification, and (4) correlation of the information to trace disease outbreaks.

Permanent identification of domestic animals has been a goal for several thousand years. Egyptian tombs dating back to 2000 B.C. show branding of livestock; Romans, Greeks, and Chinese also practiced branding in ancient times. Now, with rapid and long distance movement of animals, increased attention to animal disease prevention and needed documentation of genetic lines, animal identification is of importance to livestock culture the world over.

An ideal identification technique would be (1) permanent, (2) inexpensive, (3) easy to apply, (4) quick to apply, (5) legible at a distance of several feet, (6) painless for the animal, (7) tamper proof, (8) identify the animal individually, as well as the locale and herd, and (9) be adaptable to coding and modern data retrieval systems. These needs in large part are now being met for selected classes of animals, often of relatively high economic value and usually limited in size, and for which the various parties are in agreement on a need for identification to accomplish a specific purpose.

It is another matter to develop an ongoing system that meets all or most of the above criteria and that can be made universal and compulsory for even a single species of livestock. The largest problem is convincing livestock owners and associated interests that modern livestock production is reaching a point where required large-scale animal identification is a necessity not a luxury. It is rapidly becoming a necessity for affordable and effective animal health programs, and industry leaders know it is a key to credible long-distance marketing operations for bloodline improvement and for carcass quality control.

In the United States, one indication of the importance and difficulties of comprehensive animal identification is that the U.S. Animal Health Association (USAHA) has for many years maintained a Committee on Livestock Identification, which reports on the variety of technical methods and implementation systems that have been, or are, under study (USAHA 1972–1984). Throughout these years the committee has received reports on methods for electronic identification, including implanted transponders that can be read without close restraint of the animal. Slap tattoos for swine, of considerable interest in earlier years, lost favor for a variety of reasons, including increased use of skinning rather than dehairing at slaughter, and by 1983 the committee supported a recommendation that the slap tattoo be eliminated as an option for identification of boars in slaughter.

The fact that widely usable new identification systems have yet to be found is demonstrated by the fact that the committee has also maintained interest in upgrading specifications for ear tags, and even for glue used on back tags, in order to upgrade these familiar procedures. Recognizing that effective identification, of whatever nature, must be compulsory and enforceable was emphasized in 1984 when the committee reviewed possibilities for strengthening national regulations for interstate movement of animals to deter tampering with identification en route.

The 1984 committee report itemized some of the obstacles to national identification systems: apprehension over government interference and penalties, unreasonable tolerance levels for residues, and negative connotations of the term mandatory. All these factors act as deterrents to public acceptance of compulsory identification.

The fact that the search for new identification technology has so far not solved all the problems, that enforcement of compulsory identification needs improvement, and that there is livestock-owner resistance to mass identification does not remove the reality that more and better identification is a requisite for future progress in animal health work. The fact that the USAHA has continued to look for better animal identification for many years demonstrates the importance of this reality. Currently, the situation can be summarized as follows:

1. A variety of technologies are presently available for use in situations requiring animal identification.

2. Animal health work, including epidemiologic and trace-back studies, is so dependent on animal identification that an effective identification system must be a component of any new program if it is to succeed.

3. While the producers and processors may not yet be willing to support or accept mass compulsory animal identification, there is ample historical evidence that, if properly presented, identification will be supported for specific disease control and eradication programs, organized herd improvement programs and, in many countries, for quality control at slaughter.

4. There will be a continuing need to search for improvements in technological and operational identification procedures; ways within existing techniques must be found to convince the affected public of the necessity of identification as a component of existing and future programs.

# 15

## Operating a Disease Eradication Program

> As long as evidence for the existence of the (causative agent) continues to appear, the campaign has been a failure. There is no such thing as partial success in eradication. One either achieves glorious success or dismal failure.
>
> —F. L. SOPER, 1943

DISEASE ERADICATION PROGRAMS vary in scope depending on the range of the host animal and the infecting organism. Most eradication program efforts are carried out within a single country, but there are occasional multinational or even world programs; e.g., smallpox has recently been eradicated from the world. The campaign to eradicate the screwworm started as a regional program in the United States, but it is now a multinational program with Mexico as a cooperative participant.

Multinational programs require some system for the division of leadership. Two or more co-directors, representing different jurisdictional entities, may share responsibilities; however this arrangement can confound the best efforts of sincere and capable people unless the mix of plural bosses, laws, customs, advisory bodies, and languages, can be promptly set straight and kept that way.

This chapter discusses what is involved in programs with one director and confined to one nation.

### Program Director

A program director should not be a person who wants an even-tenored, methodical way of life. Program directors will be confronted with the vagaries of weather, capriciousness of the agent under attack, unspoken resistance, and a need to stimulate program activities that are losing momentum or to restrain those that are moving too far ahead of the total plan.

Those responsible for choosing a program director usually exercise great care in the selection process but generally are confronted with either gambling on an untested but promising individual or looking further for an experienced leader with a record of success in other programs. Since available candidates of the latter type are rare, as the rigors of working as a program director are not conducive to long tenure in that type of position, the selection of untested program administrators or directors needs to be done with great care, particularly in evaluating the nontechnical attributes of leadership as well as the often unappreciated demands of the work.

Hardships, learned through experience, are a part of program leadership, but the problems are not unique to leadership of a disease eradication effort; they beset leaders in many other fields. What is distinctive is the need to maintain constant pressure on program personnel and collaborators through years of effort. Few other leadership positions, civilian or military, require as high an energy level over such a long period. Even when the agent under attack can no longer be detected, the director must keep up the pressure for additional months or years to be sure the agent has been eliminated. To do otherwise is to risk the recrudescence of a barely surviving remnant capable, if unchallenged, of rising again to the preprogram level.

Given these realities, it is obviously immensely helpful to a field program director to have stable, honest, and intelligent supervisors who will maintain their support when the going gets rough. Fortunately, in animal health agencies led by career professionals, many agency heads have had field experience as program leaders.

Given that the pathway to final eradication will encounter formidable obstacles, there is one great consolation for the director—a singleness of purpose that enables pursuit of a clear and unmistakeable objective; contrasted with the medley of target shifts and alterations of timing and levels of effort that can be a part of a disease control program. There is seldom a concisely defined end point for control efforts, which can struggle on sporadically with short-term resources or be discontinued abruptly when support is withdrawn.

## Organizing for Action

Disease eradication programs usually start with a single plan, decided upon during the developmental process, and made final during authorization and funding. The program director, however, faces an early and difficult task in establishing the priorities of and the sequence for implementing the components of the plan. If time and resources permit, feasibility studies are helpful. Pilot programs possibly may aid in determining how best to implement the larger campaign. Results of these actions, or suggestions from interested individuals, may lead to program changes that yield welcome dividends.

Ideas for combining resources and efforts into a combined campaign to eradicate more than one disease should be rejected. It may seem efficient on superficial examination, but in reality it would be equivalent to asking a single military unit to campaign simultaneously against two enemies on two fronts.

Questions needing early assessment by a prospective or newly appointed program director are as follows:

1. Can the goal, methods of operation, and geographic limits of the projected program be defended?

2. Do the director and other individuals or groups involved understand commitments regarding the duration of assignment, duties, performance standards, unforeseen or ungovernable factors, funding, extent of authority, and intramural and extramural politics?

3. Is the line of authority clearly defined and agreed to, so that the director answers to only one superior?

4. Are there distinct, timed program phases that must be observed?

5. Are there constraints (other than judgement) to be honored regarding procedures and materials (slaughter, quarantine, vaccines, pesticides) that can be dangerous and/or controversial?

6. Is the venture a cooperative one and, if so, is there a defined and documented agreement on the division of cost, responsibility, and authority?

Beyond these questions, the director of a new program will be confronted with an array of tasks, the timing of which will vary. However, some caveats are:

1. Do not try to do everything yourself. The director cannot and should not monitor or make decisions on all details.

2. Participate decisively in the selection of key people who will be expected to get specific tasks accomplished.

3. Get the key people hired and indoctrinated as quickly as possible; explain specifically what is to be done and outline a timetable for execution.

4. Encourage the key people to work closely with one another so that their efforts mesh, important matters are not left undone, and duplication of orders or efforts is avoided.

With a planned program there is little excuse for not getting started in orderly fashion. In an emergency effort people are suddenly pulled together to face the unexpected, and there may be some hastily-contrived directions and chaotic times. However, the stress in any program, planned or emergency, should be on the initial well-timed marshalling of the key staff members and putting them to work. The director may have to step on a few toes, deviate from some procedures, or come close to breaking some administrative regulations, but personnel *can* be recruited on schedule, and supplies and equipment *can* be obtained and issued as needed.

## Staffing

The director of a disease eradication program should put great emphasis on seeking quality employees, advisors, and consultants. Culling unsuitable or incompetent people during the selection process should be as implacable at the outset as it must be later when dismissals may be necessary, for there is little margin for error during a disease eradication program. The stakes are too high and the odds of losing too great for sentimentality or compassionate gestures toward questionable candidates.

The program director establishes the pace, tone, and intensity of the campaign and is largely responsible for operational strategies and tactics. To do this properly, much effort must be devoted to counseling with the most competent colleagues and advisors. Only at great risk is reasoned, seasoned advice disregarded. Sound, lucid grounds are needed to sustain actions taken; personal whim, emotion, and bias have no place in determining action, and any change in plan deserves objective and detached examination.

Disease eradication programs, semi-permanent rather than permanent organizations, present some staffing problems unique to these types of units, particularly when coupled with the demands of the work. Competent candidates may be concerned over the (1) uncertain duration of the program, (2) increased responsibility and consequent risk of diminished career reputation, (3) missed opportunities for advancement in the more permanent, parent organization, (4) long, difficult hours that frequently characterize disease eradication work, and (5) moving the family and uprooting children in school.

It takes people of a special persuasion to forego the certainties and comforts of normal living and offer their services without reservation to an emergency disease eradication program. Yet for such programs to succeed, the key staff must be unusually competent people who are not business-as-usual types. A person anticipating selection as a director of such an effort is well advised to list the key people wanted, and informally and without commitment ascertain their willingness to serve if asked to do so later.

## Operational Leadership

The director is expected to effectively present judicious plans to persons of varied interests who must be persuaded of the soundness of the projected courses of action, often under trying circumstances. The director also must have in reserve well thought-out contingency positions that will enable compromise when serious disagreements arise. The initiative in this special arena of policy management should never be lost; to do so would be to risk loss of program momentum and orderly progress. Therefore, policy development must be a function of program leadership. In the absence of strong direction, good field employees will develop and implement their own policies. However, this can result in uneven standards and lead to valid complaints both from those affected by the program as well as from program staff.

**COMMUNICATIONS.** It is vital that each staff member and each member of the affected public knows well the goal of the program. Individuals who feel responsible for and are knowledgeable about an activity tend to understand and accept hardship better than those who feel they have not been made part of the program.

A director constantly must be prepared to provide clear, succinct, and factual briefings on the status quo. In a large program, briefings also will come from other staff members; it is important that the briefing material be communicated throughout the organization. Disparate groups must be convinced that whoever presents the material has a clear understanding of the goal of the program, knows program progress and how resources will be committed, and will respond intelligently to probing questions. This requires sincerity and sound information more than oratorical flamboyance.

The people who may be adversely affected by the program must be aggressively cultivated through respected leaders and advised of future actions and the reasons for the actions. Criticism will still result, but it is better to receive dissent from informed critics than waste time on trivial or extraneous matters stirred up by the uninformed.

Communications with the general public (see Chap. 10) often can progress beyond the usual information and education output. Specific efforts such as producer-alert systems that provide advisories when rising infection, weather favorable to the disease, or other factors that presage probable increased incidence can be shared. The crux of any public education and information effort is that a disease eradication program must deal with people as well as the pathogen, but care must be exercised and momentous events must be handled with caution and thought, even when the spurs of emergency seem to demand instant response.

For example, in the early 1950s, following two years of intensive inspection and laboratory testing, Mexico and the United States thought foot-and-mouth disease (FMD) had been eradicated from Mexico. The U.S.-Mexican border had been opened and normal livestock trade between the two countries was being reestablished. The disease reappeared on the Gulf Coast of Mexico in May 1953 (to this day no one knows why or how). United States law requires closing the U.S.-Mexican border when the disease appears in Mexico, and border officials were promptly advised to this effect from Washington, D.C. Unfortunately, this action was not coordinated with Mexican officials, even though U.S. personnel were stationed in Mexico City, working closely with Mexican officials in a joint FMD commission. News of the existence of FMD in Mexico and the border closing reached the U.S. press very quickly and that knowledge was widely disseminated before the Mexican government had an opportunity to make an official announcement to its citizens. The result was acrimonious relations between the two countries, and it was some time before rapport was reestablished in the commission and between the two governments.

**UNDERSTANDING.** Successful program leadership must have, or quickly develop, a grasp of human nature. Goals are achieved by motivated people who do things rapidly and well. Some staff will accept difficult or dangerous assignments in return for sympathetic and thoughtful words or gestures of appreciation. Some need no outside reward; their motivation stems from inner conviction and personal standards. Some individuals may be stimulated by financial reward and, if outstanding work can be prompted by money, this may have some place as an instrument for achieving goals. Unfortunately, there are still others who find concealment in the maze of an organization and may not perform at all except to avoid reprimand.

In a large organization, put together rapidly for a special purpose, it is probable that the personnel will include all these types, including the less desirable categories. In an active disease eradication program, the lazy or unmotivated have no place and should be dismissed or returned to their previous assignment. Also, be cautious in depending on those who seek added financial return in order to produce above average results. Enthusiasm, innovation, and devotion to duty can seldom be purchased. Rewards are a part of good leadership, but only for demonstrated performance. Advance promises should be avoided, for if the promised recognition fails to go through the result will be an unhappy employee.

Fortunately, disease eradication campaigns attract many outstanding people. For some the challenge is sufficient stimulus, clarity of purpose appeals to others, and some adventurous souls are happiest in the thick of the action. Most have a basic feeling that it is worthwhile to spend the extra efforts required to eradicate a harmful pathogen; it is a unique and challenging task compared to the more routine professional activities.

**SUPPLY.** Supply officers may not get much popular recognition, but even the best army cannot campaign successfully without an efficient supply system.

Supply in a large, fast-moving program is a monumental task if done well. The supply officer should have dash, enthusiasm, and initiative. As it is probable that available candidates will be new to the special demands of an eradication campaign, the person selected needs immediate indoctrination, with emphasis on tasks that must be executed with speed and accuracy. The supply officer and other staff must realize that they are as important to the goals of the program as any other part of the organization. If this is not done, the supply officer, seldom versed in biological science, may have little understanding of program operation and may adopt a routine that results in supply delays and poor field morale. Administrative personnel serve the needs of the program and the director needs to insure that no doubt exists on this point.

A multitude of paper work and regulations can throttle an otherwise aggressive program. An effective administrator finds ways to get things done and seldom takes the negative position that it cannot be done. Program supply personnel must be prepared for misunderstandings with supporting service agency sections and open-market sources of supply in regard to the (1) procurement of, and method of payment for, program materials and equipment; (2) delivery of supplies at the scheduled time and place; (3) storage, use, servicing, and legal ramifications regarding sensitive items (pesticides, nuclear materials, vaccines, special-use vehicles, and firearms are examples from U.S. programs in recent years); and (4) distribution and accountability of nonexpendable supply items.

The procedure for the purchase and delivery of diagnostic reagents, vaccines, and other critical items must insure that all the products meet high quality standards. While this may seem obvious, some of the situations that may develop in a large program that endanger such a procedure are (1) demands from higher levels for cost consciousness to the exclusion of all else (not uncommon); (2) pressures from political levels, or from cooperators, to use local sources of supply without regard to cost or quality (also not uncommon); and (3) unfortunately, occasional bribery attempts, subtle or otherwise.

If there is any doubt about the ability to ward off economic interests, politicians, or others who assume they have the power to sway decisions, the director is justified in selecting products over which such interests have no control. Ingenuity may be required, for such action frequently must be taken in a way that avoids conflict or threats of retribution to the program. Program integrity, usually arduously established over time, can be quickly eroded if these types of pressures are allowed to influence decisions.

## Strategy and Tactics

The program director must possess the patience of a starving spider and, when the opportunity arises, strike with the speed and power of a stooping falcon. A successful director husbands resources, constantly examines the logic, and makes the "big play" only when the chances are best for success or when pressing situations dictate the move. Administrative procedures can drift into a fixed routine rather than a program-oriented service function, and the program leadership must be alert that administrative regulations do not become directed toward the convenience of administrative personnel to the detriment of field units. Constant frugality is not a virtue if program personnel are deprived of sufficient funds, authority, and surveillance systems to enable determination of the optimum time for action and to carry out the action.

There is no free lunch in disease eradication. True progress is achieved by relentless and concerted application of all proven tools and techniques. Assessment (surveillance, inspection, etc.) is not an enchanting task to most people, but to the director of a program the results may be the most important product of the staff.

Well-considered innovation may provide unexpected benefits; new diagnostic aids, vaccines, or proprietary products can accelerate progress. Unusual changes in weather patterns, or in the political climate, may provide opportunities to progress faster than planned. To capitalize on such developments, program leaders must try to avoid a mind-set that rules out real consideration of anything new just because the familiar is more comfortable.

Program supervisors must regularly visit the field staff and the public affected by the campaign. Personal contact with program leaders, rather than indirect communication, is more likely to develop a sense of purpose and pride. High-level supervisors may tend to feel they cannot be spared from headquarters; however, the reality is that they cannot develop a balanced view of the campaign unless they can talk face-to-face with field personnel and see the work in progress.

One result of field visits may be to remind headquarters people of the debilitating effect of an excess of reports demanded from them. Large organizations tend to require more and more information, much of questionable utility. Reporting systems should be reviewed and pruned on a regular basis, with emphasis on measuring results, not counting activities.

Disease programs are fragile and can tolerate little tampering to suit special interests, including politicians. However, a distinction must be made between an honorable politician striving to help the general constituency and one who is an opportunist trying to exercise authority for personal or narrow partisan aims.

Honorable politicians are very important in the initiation and conduct of sound animal health programs. They are indispensable to public groups seeking funds and authority for a program and should be recognized as an essential element of program support. To be helpful, those at the political level must be knowledgeable about the concepts and procedures of the program. Program leaders should make a point of seeing that those in a position to assist program efforts are kept informed of both the achievements and the problems of the program.

An organization is seldom static and providing for orderly and qualified succession is a mark of a good administrator. However, an ancient axiom is that the messenger bringing bad tidings may lose his head. Similarly, when disaster strikes, a campaign leader may be replaced. People also retire, become ill, or move to other assignments. If the directorship is changing, a departing program director cannot expect to select a successor; that director should aim to develop qualified individuals for those in authority to consider as replacements.

## Terminating a Program

By definition, a successful disease eradication program must have an end point, which is the point at which the program can be safely terminated. A disease control program cannot truly be terminated. The most effectively operated programs are keyed to the final goal of eradication, thus, an early definition of what eradication means for the specific campaign is important.

In developing this definition, it cannot be assumed that "everyone knows" (or will admit) the meaning of eradication for a particular disease. Some may argue that eradication has been achieved when a previously prevalent disease is reduced to an occasional case; others may be satisfied with the elimination of "natural" outbreaks but balk at the idea of discontinuing vaccination; still others may feel that it is not enough to eliminate the occurrence of outbreaks, but the antibodies against the disease should also be eliminated. In terms of the general definitions in Chapter 1, the first two of these positions are not eradication but various levels of control. In contrast, the last position goes farther than normally needed and in fact will not be achievable when nonspecific antigens cause positive test results even though the agent is absent. Therefore, the definition needs to be more than just the words eradication or control; it needs to be specifically stated in terms of the particular agent targeted.

As eradication is absolute rather than relative, there must be a specified end point. Once conditions are met that satisfy the stated goal, the program as well as the disease is ended.

A control program is never ended if gains made are to be protected. Although it may be possible to define the level of control desired before a continuing maintenance level is instituted, a valid definition of the end point for a control program cannot include a statement, or implication, that no further efforts will be required.

End-point definition is also an important means of maintaining support for an eradication program during a difficult period, the time after the disease seems to have disappeared and before it can be finally determined that it is truly eradicated. During this period extensive and expensive searches for any residual infection are necessary. Since the disease is no longer obvious, appropriation requests for this type of search are almost always challenged as unnecessary unless it can be demonstrated that the final surveillance period is not only an essential part of the total program but has been a defined part of the program since its inception.

**PROCEDURES.** There are three primary factors to be satisfied before an eradication program can be credibly terminated: (1) the "last case" must be clearly established as having in fact been the final occurrence of the disease, (2) other means for future internal spread must be identified and neutralized, and (3) any special barriers needed to prevent reintroduction must be in place. As no one can identify the last case at the time it is found and eliminated, it must be defined by a surveillance program carried out for a long enough period to withstand an objective review.

Post-disease surveillance should continue at whatever level necessary to locate outbreaks during the final stages: survey inspections, screen testing, mandatory reporting, or some combination of these. Final surveillance involves the same activities, with continuing laboratory support appropriate for the particular program. If final surveillance depends primarily on inspection or screen testing, the survey pattern should be comprehensive enough to provide results that are representative of the disease status of the target population. Surveillance that depends on reporting of suspicious illness cannot be structured in this fashion. It needs to be continually publicized to maintain a volume of suspicious reports large enough to give confidence that the disease, if present, would be identified.

The length of time that final surveillance should be maintained depends on the characteristics of the disease and cycles of spread identified during the program. If transmission is frequently associated with the reproduction cycle, the surveillance period should cover at least two such cycles. The same principle applies to programs against diseases that historically have spread during peak marketing periods. Diseases that develop slowly, or have multiple means of transmission, may require a surveillance period of several years before there is an acceptable level of confidence that eradication has been achieved.

An example of final surveillance through inspection was the concluding stages of the sheep scabies (psoroptic) eradication program in the United States. Previously endemic states organized statewide mass inspection of all sheep, starting on a fixed date and continuing until completed. Inspection cycles were timed to follow periods of likely exposure due to leasing of rams or other farm-to-farm transfers, direct or through markets.

Screen testing alone, while a key factor in reducing initial levels of infection for diseases such as brucellosis or tuberculosis, cannot be expected to suffice for final surveillance. General population surveys must cover a large percentage of the high-risk population to give representative results, and are consequently very costly. If nonspecific antigens are present when the target agent is approaching extinction, trace-back time will be wasted in tracking false leads; therefore, for most programs final surveillance is a combination of search techniques. Screen testing can be useful if confined to the highest risk elements of the general population. Statewide freedom from bovine tuberculosis, for example, is determined through a system of slaughterhouse monitoring for suspicious lesions, laboratory analysis, trace-back procedures, and selective tuberculin testing. Five years of such efforts, with no evidence of the disease, is currently required in the United States.

For eradication programs that are primarily dependent on field reporting of suspect cases to locate infection (screwworms or hog cholera), a high level of suspicious reports must be sought and maintained during the final period, with none of these being confirmed on investigation. In the case of hog cholera in the United States, 778 suspicious reports were received and investigated during the last full calendar year between the last case and the declaration of eradication. None of these were confirmed. The 18 months (1 August 1976 to 31 January 1978) of active surveillance between the last case and the declaration of eradication included three breeding and marketing cycles.

Before termination of the program, it is also important to locate and neutralize other potential means of internal spread. Seed stocks of the agent should be allowed only in rigidly controlled, high-security facilities where such stocks are required for research, reference, or diagnostic purposes. Most research or diagnostic facilities, as well as biologics producers, are not equipped to retain an exotic disease agent, have no necessity to do so, and should not have the responsibility for preventing escape of the agent from the facility. Living-agent vaccines, as well as seed stock for vaccine production, are in the same category.

Maintenance of measures to prevent reintroduction are also required. In addition to the obvious need for either prohibition or tight restriction over importation of animals or products capable of carrying the disease, other measures may be needed. Maintenance of a barrier zone along borders with an adjacent infected country is an additional protective device used by some countries, which may require removing all susceptible domestic animals from the zone and supplementing this with a patrol system for detecting illegal introductions. Slaughterhouse sampling of animals from areas of high risk of exposure can also be utilized.

It is important, for financial and other resource utilization reasons, to terminate an eradication program as soon as possible; it is also important to maintain a credible effort to find the disease until a declaration of eradication can be made with confidence that it will withstand critical examination. This is necessary not only to insure against resurgence of the disease but also to provide a sound basis for requesting removal of prohibitions or restrictions previously imposed by other countries.

# 16

# Role of the
# Private Practitioner

THE VETERINARIAN ENGAGED in private practice, while not primarily dependent on official duties for professional activity or income, must at times carry out public responsibilities required by laws and regulations. This official role is important not only to the practitioner's clientele, but also to the work of the animal health agencies.

For the large animal practitioner, success will be measured by an ability to protect or increase the clients' income. Professionally, the work is generally with the individual animal, herd, or flock. The government animal health agency is primarily concerned with protection of the total population, and the laws that the agency administers are written to protect the general society.

Most animal disease programs, no matter how carefully structured to protect the rights and economic interests of the individual owners, cause hardship for some. The practitioner with a personal and economic relationship with a client can be caught between that client who feels adversely affected by official requirements and the responsibility as a licensed professional to serve the public interest. The public service veterinarian faces this type of conflict only when political pressure is exerted on behalf of an owner seeking an exception to regulatory requirements.

Yet the private and public segments of the profession must mutually carry out joint tasks. Usually, it is not possible, or desirable, for government staff to provide all the official functions needed in the field, including preparing and certifying animals for sale or shipment or meeting the personnel demands needed in a large disease control or eradication program. As urbanization and industrialization of society has increased, the emphasis in veterinary service has shifted away from large animal practice, reducing the proportion of veterinarians engaged in food animal medicine and increasing the need for effective utilization of those remaining.

## General Veterinary Practice Activity

Prior to World War I the primary veterinary activity in the United States was caring for the working equine, as it was in other countries with similar societies. By the 1980s most practitioners in the United States were working primarily with small animals; the draft horse and mule had largely disappeared, and the modern equine practitioner was concerned with pleasure and racing animals.

The extent of this change is shown in data on the division of veterinary activity and domestic animal populations (AVMA 1983). Only one out of three veterinary practitioners was engaged, exclusively or in part, in food animal medicine. Most of the balance (64%) were predominantly in small animal practice, and 4% were identified as equine practitioners. Of the approximately one in four U.S. veterinarians not engaged in private practice, it is the estimate of the authors, based on personal work experience, that not more than 15% of these are employed by federal and state animal health agencies. This leads to the conclusion that currently only about 28% of the active veterinarians in the United States are working directly with the health of food animals at the farm or ranch level.

When related to the animal population, this means that direct veterinary support for livestock production is spread more thinly than for other segments of the animal population: 107 million small animals (1983), 8 million horses (1983), and 185 million cattle, swine, and sheep (1982). There is now about one equine practitioner for every 6500 horses; one small animal practitioner for every 6100 small animals; but only one veterinarian, public or private, for every 20,500 food animals, not including poultry, an industry that has required several large-scale disease eradication programs in recent years.

Animal health agencies do not have sufficient veterinary staffing to meet either ongoing or emergency disease prevention needs alone; therefore, those veterinary practitioners still engaged in food animal medicine are of increasing importance to the work of these agencies. A structured system for utilizing private practitioners in official animal health activities is a necessity.

## Practitioner Certification for Official Work

Veterinary education is necessarily directed toward preparing graduates for private practice, and it is these private practitioners, food animal practitioners in particular, who are often called upon to carry out professional work required by laws and regulations. This ranges from the required reporting of certain diseases; health examination, testing, and inoculations required for sale or shipment; veterinary inspection at marketing points; to, on occasion, contract work for animal health agencies in control and eradication programs.

In these official activities the practitioner is primarily a representative of the public—a role that requires an emphasis and understanding sufficiently different from the usual practice demands to require orientation and training at a level not fully covered in the usual veterinary education.

In the United States the certification of practitioners for official work is called accreditation, a formal process in addition to satisfying the requirements for a degree in veterinary medicine and for licensure by a state examining board.

Accreditation procedures, included in the United States Code of Federal Regulations, require certification by state and federal animal health authorities that the practitioner is not only a qualified professional but has received training in official work and responsibilities. Only accredited veterinarians can legally issue certificates required by animal health regulations and perform other official work required by such regulations. Loss of accreditation means loss of the legal authority to do this work for official purposes. Therefore, it is in the interest of the veterinarian, as well as the clients, to maintain accredited status.

From the standpoint of the public animal health agencies, the accredited veterinarian brings unique benefits to official animal health responsibilities:

1. Practitioners are readily available to the livestock owner for consultation. Owners look to practitioners as a source of program information and professional advice.

2. Practitioners provide an early warning network for detecting diseases dangerous to the public good; early detection and reporting can mean the difference between success or failure in disease eradication.

3. Practitioners know the management practices of owners in their practice area.

4. Practitioners are respected by their clients, and their advice and recommendations are viewed with more confidence than those of outsiders.

5. Practitioners often are the only liaison between the owner and the animal health agency, and a practitioner's evaluation of a program is important to the owner.

6. Practitioners are a source of professional staffing to augment government personnel in large-scale animal health programs. This can lower total program cost, provide wider and faster program coverage, and improve owner cooperation.

## Building Sound Relationships

There are certain duties and responsibilities in practitioner–health agency working relationships that need to be understood and met by each party. Government agencies have the responsibility for carrying out public programs to protect animal health and are obligated to take the initiative in organizing and administering the effort.

Responsibilities for the agency include the following:

1. Provide liaison and curriculum assistance to veterinary colleges to lay a foundation in public veterinary service philosophy and operations as part of classroom instruction, including emphasis on the ethics and obligations of public service.

2. Maintain a certification or accreditation process that will equip the practitioner with the procedures required and the rationale for such procedures.

3. Maintain a follow-up process after certification that will not only cover changes in procedures but include full reports on, and analysis of, operational animal health programs.

4. Maintain, through field veterinary staff, personal contact with veterinary practitioners to enable interchange of ideas and questions and to monitor the effectiveness of the work being performed.

5. Utilize veterinarians contracted for field services as professionals equivalent to full-time staff, providing them with the same background information and holding them to the same standards of performance.

6. Maintain the integrity of accreditation by acting decisively to remove approval from individuals unwilling or unable to maintain required standards.

7. Encourage veterinary staff at national, state, and local levels to actively participate in professional associations.

Responsibilities for the accredited veterinarian include the following:

1. Keep informed on general regulatory requirements and the progress of programs in active operation.

2. When carrying out official work, operate as a professional rather than as a technician, which includes discussing with the owner what is being done, why it is necessary, how it fits into the program, the goals of the program, and what the owner can expect from the program.

3. Recognize that all official work, whether paid for by the owner or through contract fees from public sources, is as much a part of a complete veterinary practice as any other professional activity and deserves the same level of service.

4. If circumstances arise that the practitioner is not equipped to handle, call for support rather than attempt to develop an answer or an action that may be incorrect.

The private practitioner performing official work faces relationship conflicts not usually encountered by the public service veterinarian. It takes a self-disciplined practitioner possessed with a high degree of professionalism to maintain the correct course of action in such circumstances. The importance of the private practitioner to the total animal health effort is such that the practitioner deserves full support and recognition from the public agencies.

# 17

# Task Forces

MOST PREPLANNED DISEASE CONTROL and eradication campaigns are handled through the existing field organization. Field staff may be expanded, specialized technical assistance added, and administrative support enlarged, but the established framework remains the basis for the work. Permanent field supervisors know the peculiarities of the local environment and how to get things done under local conditions.

On occasion, however, this ongoing structure, no matter how effective it has been in meeting previous assignments, may be presented with a challenge beyond its capacity. This usually happens with the introduction of a new and potentially explosive disease, or from the emergence of an epidemic of an existing disease for which a program is underway. The use of a special task force may be the most effective way to resolve the problem quickly and completely.

In health program work, a task force is a tactical unit drawn from several sources and assigned to execute a specific mission. The force is a temporary grouping, under one leader, directed to solve a defined disease problem that requires a saturation effort beyond the capacity of the local field organization.

While the specifics of future problems are not predictable, the types of skills generally required can be a part of advanced contingency planning. Qualified people can be put on a standby table of organization. A group of qualified specialists, selected and trained in advance, can surround and eliminate a disease problem more effectively than a group thrown together hastily in response to an unanticipated emergency. Through preselection and pretraining, those chosen learn the types of problems they would encounter in the field and their general responsibilities if called upon. A better understanding will result if periodic opportunity is provided to participate in test exercises simulating anticipated field problems. Preselection also provides time for the supervisors of those selected to know of, and agree to, the assignment. Administrative procedures relating to travel and compensation can also be established in advance.

130

## Activation

A properly staffed and supported task force can produce results, but it is also expensive. A decision to activate this type of operation is not one to be made casually. The technical questions to be examined are

1. In the case of an existing program, is it known why the disease has grown locally to epidemic proportions?
2. In the case of a new disease, is enough known about how the disease should be handled to predict with some confidence that the outbreak can be contained and eliminated?

Some management considerations are

1. Do the resident field people have the required numbers, experience, and initiative?
2. If not, can changes in leadership or expansion of skills and numbers be expected to solve the problem?
3. Are existing administrative facilities and capabilities adequate to handle the additional load?

If the answers to the technical questions are affirmative but the management considerations produce doubt about the ability to do the work required, activation of a task force may offer the best hope for success. A common error made by administrators is to delay creation of a task force in order to give the local field organization an opportunity to solve the problem. Usually this results from a feeling (probably correct) that local personnel will be unhappy if outsiders are brought in and a desire to avoid the added expense.

Delay can be a mistake. The greatest benefit from a task force is an early and large-scale attack when drastic action is needed. Although the money, personnel, and materials must be found, the potential expense should not be cause for delay if there is rapid deterioration of a program in the field or if there is an introduction of a new and dangerous disease.

A new group may provide the quickest results because a permanent field group is accustomed to working in familiar patterns at expected levels of effort; their working relationships have been established. For ongoing programs requiring cooperation between several political jurisdictions or agencies, areas of compromise have developed to keep the work going. It is often difficult to alter these work patterns and relationships rapidly enough when a large new problem appears. If the problem gets out of hand and threatens to overwhelm the local field force (which is not unusual), a new force under new command, with no prior commitments, can work at a level of urgency not previously possible.

Effective operation of a task force is dependent on rapid exercise of administrative effort with a fresh viewpoint. For most operations office space, living quarters, and communication capabilities are needed immediately, as are vehicles and other material support. This level of support usually cannot be met by existing local facilities or supplies, and the customary procurement procedures are too slow.

## Organization and Operation

Single command is so important for successful task force operation that it should be considered a prerequisite; therefore, the selection of the task force director is of great significance. Experience, good judgment, and leadership are required, and the director must be able to work under sustained pressure and delegate authority. A task force operation can be expected to involve a variety of interests, thus the director must also have the political skill to keep all the parties working toward the objective.

Since the task force moves into an area during a deteriorating field situation, usually when emotions are running high, it is essential to clearly establish the unchallenged leadership authority of the director. The task force director should not be confronted with interagency conflict; assignment of personnel, allotment of funds, and interagency jurisdictional questions must be settled at levels above the task force itself.

Task force staffing will vary in size and diversity according to the nature and scope of the problem. Divisions of function include field operations, administrative support, and a technical staff to carry out laboratory support, evaluation and analysis, and planning. Any problem of sufficient importance to warrant use of a task force will also attract attention from the news media; therefore, it is advantageous to have a capable, experienced information officer, who will not only save the director a great deal of time but also will keep others in the organization from being pursued by reporters.

While the field operations group of the task force is involved with the usual activities associated with health programs, the level of effort is not that of the usual program: a task force operation is a saturation effort done as quickly as possible. The field operations people need to be able to organize their time well and should not be overly concerned about normal working hours. They should be self-starters capable of working independently, particularly if the area is large and it is necessary to establish suboffices to avoid excessive travel time.

The technical staff is tailored to the problem: those selected for these assignments not only must be qualified in their specialty but must be able to work within short time frames and be willing to spend a lot of time in the field.

Experience has demonstrated the need for a field epidemiologist as part of this team. Rapid diagnosis is also essential, and if laboratory support is required, a field laboratory should be established if possible.

Needed expertise should be sought wherever it exists, which frequently means going outside the agency conducting the program. Entomologists expert in wide-area application of pesticides and use of aircraft in vector control can be found in agricultural agencies responsible for plant protection programs. Military medical support units may be able to assist with laboratory personnel. Noncommissioned officers from the military can supervise quarantine lines and disinfection stations.

Advisors to the staff may be needed in other specialized areas, such as wildlife management, marketing, the disease under attack, and meat or poultry inspection. Initially, going outside the program agency may take some vision on the part of the task force director or agency superiors, but once the worth of outside advisors or staff specialists has been demonstrated, it will be quickly sought on subsequent occasions.

The organization for the type of task force used in the United States is shown in Figure 17.1. The depth of assignments shown may not be required in all cases, but each position has been found necessary in one or more operations. This arrangement, one for each of five geographic regions in the United States, has been tested under actual disease emergencies involving several dis-

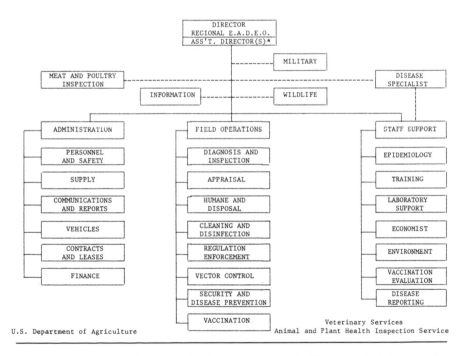

**Fig. 17.1.** Organization pattern for the regional emergency disease eradication task forces. *State official(s), depending on the state(s) involved in the outbreak. (USDA Regional Emergency Animal Disease Eradication Organizations administrative publication)

eases, several species, and several geographic locations and is the outgrowth of operational experience developed during the 1970s. The use of task forces in the United States during these years benefited from similar operations conducted in special situations during the Mexican-U.S. foot-and-mouth disease eradication program in the 1950s.

The essential characteristic of a successful task force, whether small or large, is a sense of urgency. Events move rapidly; review and analysis are constant and operational plans are frequently revised. Communication can become a problem, and daily briefings involving the director and staff are usually required to discuss policy and coordinate efforts. If the operation becomes routine the purpose is lost.

Experience has demonstrated the value of timely use of a task force of sufficient size and experience. Difficulties are usually due to delay in activating the unit, insufficient financial support, or the choice of a director not suited to this type of operation.

# 18

# Wildlife

To MOST PEOPLE, the term wildlife conjures up visions
of a group of mammalian game animals and furbearers. These species certainly
are wildlife, but many others including rodent, avian, reptilian, arthropod,
and amphibian members also should be considered. Members of these species
are present in, or close to, nearly every human and domestic animal community. This propinquity, their large numbers, and their susceptibility to pathogens of other species suggests that wild species are likely to be involved in many
transmission cycles and influence many control or eradication programs.

One of the classic examples of wildlife involvement in livestock disease
cycles occurred in Kenya in 1909, when African swine fever was recognized,
described, and differentiated from hog cholera (Montgomery 1921). The disease broke out on farms where wart hogs (*Phacochoerus*) and bush pigs (*Poto-
machoerus*) were found. It was later demonstrated that these species are inapparent carriers of the virus.

More recently identified examples involving wildlife as important reservoirs for pathogens of other species include small mammals in Rocky Mountain
spotted fever; raccoons, squirrels, skunks, and mice in leptospirosis; numerous
reptiles and amphibia in salmonellosis; and many avian species in arboviral
encephalitides.

In other instances, wildlife appear to be incidental rather than the maintaining hosts, i.e., they are occasionally infected from, but unlikely to be a
source for, other species. An example of this is *Brucella abortus* in the white-
tailed deer. In the early years of the bovine brucellosis eradication program,
many dairy farmers in the eastern United States were convinced that the deer
often observed in their pastures were responsible for perpetuating the disease
in their herds. Some states issued special permits to dairy farmers to shoot such
deer as a disease control measure.

Numerous subsequent surveys have not demonstrated any evidence of
significant involvement of white-tailed deer in brucellosis transmission (Moore
and Schnurrenberger 1981). In retrospect, this lack of involvement is understandable despite their susceptibility. Does are solitary during fawning season,

when risk of spreading brucellae to cattle could be expected to be greatest, and drop their fawns in wooded areas rather than open pastures frequented by cattle. Also, deer normally do not graze on pastures, except in early spring; they feed on wood browse and acorns and usually are seen in pastures while moving from one part of their range to another. They have different habits than, and do not closely associate with, cattle.

It is obvious from these examples that the potential role of wildlife must be considered in planning a control or eradication program. Contingency plans for programs to be initiated in the event an exotic disease agent is introduced must include determination of whether or not indigenous wild species can be infected by and transmit the organism. Information, if it exists, will have to be found in countries where the pathogen is present or under extremely secure conditions. As with most aspects of any specific regulatory program, however, no generalizations can be drawn that will necessarily apply to another disease agent or another geographic area.

Planning a program against an already established pathogen must include the possibility of wild species involvement and whether or not the agent has already infected this population. It is evident that an eradication scheme for an agent in domestic animals may be compromised if the pathogen is present in the wild population, e.g., rabies.

In countries where rabies is already present in many wild species (as in the Americas), eradication in domestic species is not feasible and control measures are the only practical approach. In island areas or countries where rabies is not present in wild or domestic species (Australia, Great Britain, Hawaii), the aim is to keep the disease out of wild animals by rigid import procedures for domestic animals. If an eradication program is contemplated against an existing agent and adequate, reliable information on the situation in susceptible wild species is not available, studies should be considered. When planning for the hog cholera eradication program in the United States, several uncertainties were encountered that illustrate this situation.

Research had shown that under laboratory conditions hog cholera virus (HCV) could be transmitted from pig to pig by the swine lungworm. Since the the earthworm is the intermediate host in the life cycle of the lungworm, another wild species was brought into the equation. Laboratory studies also had shown that the raccoon could carry latent HCV that could revert to pathogenicity in pigs under stress. Those opposed to the initiation of the program postulated that hog cholera eradication would not be possible in the United States due to perpetuation of the virus in species outside domestic swine.

However, Canada also had lungworms, earthworms, and raccoons and had successfully stamped out hog cholera for 50 years by concentrating on domestic swine; therefore it was decided not to be concerned about these possible modes of transmission under field conditions.

Though there was no concern about the white-collared peccary (research had shown that HCV in peccaries died out quite rapidly), there was concern about the possible threat wild swine (descendants of European wild boars originally brought into private game preserves and domestic pigs gone wild, which roamed along the South Atlantic and Gulf coasts) might pose to successful eradication. Could there possibly be an inapparent carrier status in these wild populations?

Fortunately, the Southeastern Cooperative Wildlife Disease Study (SCWDS) determined that European wild boars and feral pigs were as subject to illness and death from HCV as were domestic swine. The decision was that while these populations posed a potential risk, there was not sufficient cause to abandon the projected eradication program.

During the program, there was one incident of HCV spreading to feral pigs in northern Florida that took several months to eliminate by trapping. Later in the program it was found that insufficient attention had been given to virus transmission by insects, although there had been reports of this in earlier literature. Additional studies on insect transmission resulted in modifications to the field program in some infected areas during the latter years of the program.

This history illustrates that even though a great deal of information was available for program planning, it still was necessary to initiate additional work on the role of wildlife prior to and during the program.

A relatively ordered approach may not be possible with the sudden advent of a previously exotic pathogen that requires immediate response. In such a situation during eradication efforts, wildlife studies may be needed to decide on proper courses of action. Two such instances have occurred in the United States in recent years, both involving introduction of previously exotic agents into domestic fowl.

In the early 1960s duck virus enteritis appeared in a large concentration of domestic ducks on Long Island, New York. The initial eradication program, organized along classic lines, was altered to one of disease control after it was found that the virus was already present in migratory waterfowl.

In the early 1970s viscerotropic velogenic Newcastle disease (VVND) virus was introduced into domestic chickens in southern California and was attacked with a massive eradication campaign. It was evident that if the virus had also entered the free-flying wild bird population, successful eradication was questionable and spread from coast to coast seemed likely. The SCWDS collected over 13,800 potentially free-ranging domestic or wild birds from sites designated as high-risk areas. Early in this surveillance program, information obtained strongly suggested that if free-flying birds were involved in the spread of VVND, they were of the domestic type, and corrective measures were immediately inaugurated.

Of 9446 wild birds processed, VVND virus was isolated from only 3 of 1817 house sparrows and 1 crow of 472 collected. All sparrow and crow virus isolations were from infected premises where maximum exposure had occurred, and two of the three sparrows were from a single premise where heavy chicken mortality was being experienced; the crow was known to ingest chicken eggs. No VVND virus was isolated from mourning doves, starlings, migratory ducks and geese, and numerous other wild bird species that probably had been exposed to infected poultry (USDA 1978).

The conclusion is that it is a prudent regulatory policy to recognize the potential impact of wildlife in program planning and execution and to gather the maximum amount of information possible before making decisions. But the impact of wildlife on a program is only one side of the equation; the potential impact of a control or eradication program on wildlife is also involved.

National and international political realities require that we be aware of the impact of our programs on the total environment. Strong worldwide interest in protecting endangered species, removing or reducing man-made contaminants from the environment, and the growing realization that we have the ability to destroy as well as create, will make concern for wildlife even more important in the future.

Domestic animal disease programs can affect wildlife due to deliberate program policy or from indirect alteration of the existing balance of nature brought about by the programs. Two programs in the United States illustrate these possibilities.

In February 1924, foot-and-mouth disease (FMD) virus entered central California through garbage from a naval shipyard near San Francisco. By summer it had spread south and east into the cattle and sheep ranges in a national forest.

In July a cattle rancher with an infected herd found lesions of the disease in dead deer on his leased range in the forest. A survey showed deer on other ranges were infected, thus a deer reduction program utilizing shooting and poisoning was implemented in the fall when the deer were driven down to lower elevations by cold weather.

The deer reduction effort was ended the following June after no more active infection was found in deer; hunting crews had taken 20,819 deer, with observed infection rates varying from 24% at the beginning of the hunt to 0% at the end.

This drastic impact on the deer population in one national forest resulted from direct action taken to support an eradication program to protect domestic livestock. It was successful, and the grazing areas were restocked with cattle and sheep after a 1-yr vacation period. However, public opposition to the deer kill was high, and at one point the hunting parties had to be withdrawn for fear of mob violence. The U.S. Secretary of Agriculture finally stationed a personal representative in the area for several months to obtain cooperation and allow completion of the program. That was over 50 years ago; public sensitivity in the United States would be much greater today.

Eradication programs against domestic animal disease agents also can have beneficial effects on wildlife. Eradication of the screwworm fly from the United States during the last 20 years has not only brought great benefits to livestock producers in the southeast and southwest but also has altered the size of wild populations. Deer populations have risen dramatically in many areas as the survival rate of fawns has increased, presumably because they no longer are killed from umbilical infestation by screwworm larvae. As prey animal populations have increased and their range expanded, so have the numbers of predators such as coyotes. The preprogram balance of nature has been changed and a new balance established at denser population levels as a result of the screwworm eradication program.

The role of wildlife in a specific livestock disease situation is not always permanent. Program officials must be alert for, and responsive to, changes such as occurred in New Zealand's bovine tuberculosis eradication campaign (Adlam 1979). The agent, *Mycobacterium bovis,* had not been detected in other hosts until a dramatic increase in the population of opossums resulted in a depletion of their preferred foods, forcing them into pastures frequented by cattle. The opossums now appear to be involved in maintaining the pathogen.

General questions that should be asked in relation to wildlife when considering a plan of action are

1. What wildlife species are present in the area?
2. How large is the wild population?
3. Is there contact between wild and domestic animals?
4. What is known about the ranging and feeding habits of the wild species?
5. Can the pathogen exist in wild species indigenous to the area?
6. If so, does disease appear in such wild species?
7. Do the wild species shed the agent in numbers and in a manner likely to infect livestock?
8. After considering the information available to answer these questions, is it prudent to proceed with the program?

The questions are valid; however, the information needed to provide answers may be scarce or difficult to interpret. Regulatory veterinarians, including program planners, are seldom equipped to either gather or fully understand the information that may be available. They will save time and trouble by consulting wildlife specialists who are familiar with local conditions and knowledgeable of the regional fauna and interaction with domestic species.

Evaluation of wildlife risk depends in part on the ranging and feeding habits of the wild species involved. A pertinent example has already been mentioned, that of duck virus enteritis. Since some migrating waterfowl that often congregate to feed in association with domestic ducks carry the virus, it is probably no coincidence that in the United States the disease was first observed in the domestic flocks located in the eastern flyway. In addition to the species capable of moving between countries and continents, the ranging and feeding habits of wild mammals can also affect the level of risk to a disease eradication program.

Local wildlife density can be critical to the movement of disease agents back and forth between domestic and wild animals. In areas where susceptible wild species have been hunted or driven out prior to initiating a pathogen eradication program, there may be little need for concern about risk from wildlife. However, large wildlife populations pose greater risks and require more effort, as illustrated by the effect of the increased deer population in the eastern United States.

At the turn of the century the population of the Virginia white-tailed deer had been hunted down to negligible numbers. With game management and restocking programs, the population has rapidly grown to where there are millions of deer east of the Mississippi River and, in some states, the numbers approach the size of the domestic cattle population. This large, susceptible wild population must now be reckoned with when planning for handling any future introduction of FMD virus.

In contrast to the relatively plentiful amount of data available on the habits and habitats of wildlife, it is probable that limited information will be available on their susceptibility and responses to a particular disease agent. Often, there is a scarcity of data on the pertinent epidemiologic questions relating to shedding: portals, duration, and quantity. These items, coupled with ecologic interaction with domestic species, define the probability that transmission will occur.

The importance of studying pathogen crossover from wild to domestic animals is demonstrated by a series of research studies on the origin of the virus causing vesicular exanthema of swine. This disease, and the successful campaign to eradicate it from U.S. swine, was briefly reviewed in Chapter 4. It appeared in garbage-fed swine in California in 1932, eventually (1952) moved into most states, and was stamped out in 1956. Even though the disease was eliminated from the United States, the origin of the virus was not known. The disease has, to date, not been reported in swine in any other country. Where was the reservoir?

In 1972 a virus was isolated from sea lions that caused abortion and vesicular lesions in these animals. First called San Miguel sea lion virus, subsequent study showed its relationship to the virus causing vesicular exanthema of swine. Further research led to a conclusion that there is a variety of types of caliciviruses, which involve swine and several seal species, that cannot be differentiated in swine. The virus also can be found in opaleye fish, which may serve as a primary ocean reservoir, and five species of Pacific whales (Smith 1984).

An obvious hypothesis is that the initial source of the virus in California swine fed uncooked garbage was in marine animals, either fish or mammals. It is further obvious that ecologic separation cannot forever prevent a future crossover and that such marine species should not be fed to swine.

Thought must be given to this interrelationship of wild and domestic animal populations if they coexist in an area to be subjected to a disease control or eradication effort. This cannot be done effectively without the expertise of wildlife specialists. Furthermore, wildlife species, habits, and general environmental conditions vary widely between geographic areas, and wildlife specialists who have knowledge of local conditions must be sought out.

In addition to the technical information needed from these professionals, there may be strong political considerations for including wildlife agencies in program planning and management. In many countries the wild population is not only a publicly owned resource but also an increasingly important source of revenue. In many societies there is a deep and growing attachment to the preservation of wildlife.

Regulatory veterinarians and allied livestock and poultry interests normally do not have either the technical knowledge or the type of political expertise to properly evaluate the relationship of wildlife and wildlife interests to their programs. Therefore, they usually cannot devise a plan of action that will meld the needs of the program and the concerns of those primarily interested in wildlife. Rather than wait for problems to develop, program planners should strive to develop early liaison with wildlife management agencies so the goals and responsibilities of the two interest areas can be discussed, common goals and needs identified, and a base of mutual understanding arrived at.

In the United States, basic national responsibility for the welfare of domestic animals belongs to the U.S. Department of Agriculture in collaboration with the states, but responsibility for the welfare of wildlife is divided between state and federal wildlife management agencies. Coping with jurisdictional problems is difficult for any single state or federal agency. Not all problems can be anticipated, but with prior mutual discussion many can be reduced to a level that will serve domestic livestock and wildlife interests alike. An example of cooperative efforts occurred in 1979 when 49 out of 50 state game and fish agencies and over 5000 trained personnel participated in a test exercise by the U.S. Department of Agriculture for combating a hypothetical introduction of FMD virus.

# 19

# Arthropods, Arthropod-borne Diseases, and Their Control

ARTHROPODS, invertebrate animals having jointed legs, chitinous exoskeletons, and segmented body parts, include insects, spiders, and crabs. Arthropod-borne diseases comprise an epidemiologically distinct group of infections with unique seasonal and geographic patterns. Control problems are determined by the mode of transmission of the pathogen; when the arthropod is also the reservoir, herd immunity will not operate in the host species. Other important vector characteristics are frequency of feeding, length of life, duration of infectivity, host preference, home range, and dispersal method. Arthropods that feed frequently from multiple hosts are more likely to become infected and serve as sources for new hosts. Long-lived vectors (those that can survive long periods without feeding) and multiple-host ticks present special control problems. Host preference also determines, to a great extent, the species that will suffer from certain diseases. The geographic distribution and home range of arthropods, their methods of dispersal, their infection rate, their immune status, and the density of their hosts combine to produce the disease incidence.

## Important Arthropod Pests, Vectors, and Diseases

**TICKS.** These arthropods are principally pests of horses and range cattle. The Gulf Coast tick (*Amblyomma maculatum*) and the lone star tick (*A. americanum*) are the most common in the southeastern United States, the Rocky Mountain spotted fever tick (*Dermacentor andersoni*) is prevalent in the western United States, the brown dog tick (*D. variabilis*) affects animals in the central and eastern states, and the spinose ear tick (*Octobius megnini*) troubles many types of animals in the warmer climates of the United States. In the United States ticks have served as vectors of Q fever, piroplasmosis (Texas fever or redwater fever), anaplasmosis, and Western equine encephalitis. Heavy infestations of ticks can weaken cattle and directly contribute to weight losses or even death. Fowl ticks in poultry houses can disrupt laying and weaken heavily parasitized birds.

**MITES.** Different species of mange and scab mites (*Psoroptes, Sarcoptes, Chorioptes, Psorergates, Demodex, Dermanyssus,* and *Liponyssus*) attack horses, swine, cattle, sheep, and fowl. These species are both burrowing and surface feeders, can cause skin lesions through severe skin irritation, and are almost too small to be seen with the naked eye.

**FLIES.** Both the immature (maggot) stages and the adult stages of flies are important pests of livestock. In the United States the species include the warble or heel flies (*Hypoderma bovis* and *H. lineatum*). Three species of horse botflies (*Gastrophilus intestinalis, G. nasalis,* and *G. haemorrhoidalis*) cause itching, lowered vitality, colic, and annoyance and panic among horses. Horn flies (*Siphona irritans*) cause restlessness and loss of appetite and vitality (due to blood loss) among cattle. They generally are not disease transmitters because they remain almost constantly associated with one animal. Stable flies, or dog flies (*Stomoxys calcitrans*), are also annoying pests and can serve as transmitters of anthrax bacillus and equine encephalitis virus. Face flies (*Musca autumnalis*) were first detected in the United States in 1953 and have spread rapidly. Their importance is due to the large populations that accumulate on animals, causing irritation by feeding on secretions around the sensitive areas of eyes and muzzle. Face flies affect cattle, horses, and also sheep in some areas. Horse flies (*Tabanus* spp.) and deer flies (*Chrysops* spp.) are vicious biters of cattle and equines and can cause severe blood loss, weight loss, or serve as vectors of *Anaplasma* or *Bacillus anthracis*.

The sheep botfly (*Oestrus ovis*) is a nasal fly that causes severe infestations, often accompanied by bacterial infection, causing "snotty nose." Larval infestations can interfere with feeding and may cause death due to suffocation. Sheep keds (*Melophagus ovinus*) are wingless flies that live in the fleece of sheep, feed on blood, and may cause weight loss, reduced disease resistance, general unthriftiness, and decreased growth of wool fibers. In the United States the blue-black fly (*Phormia regina*) causes "strike" among sheep, especially in damp wool soiled by feces or urine.

**LICE.** There are two types of lice: sucking lice (*Anoplura*), which are all mammalian parasites and biting lice (*Mallophaga*), which have adapted to both birds and mammals. Lice are very host specific. Cattle lice include the cattle-biting louse (*Bovicola bovis*), the sucking short-nosed cattle louse (*Haematopinus eurysternus*), the tail louse (*H. Quadripertusus*), the long-nosed or blue louse (*Linognathus vituli*), and the small blue or capillate louse (*Solenopotes* capillatus). There is only a single species of hog louse (*Haematopinis suis*). The horse-biting louse (*Trichodectes equi*) and the horse-sucking louse (*Haematopinus asini*) usually are most prevalent on the head, neck, withers, and base of the tail of equines. Lice of sheep and goats (*Trichodectes* spp., *Bovicola* spp., and *Linognathus* spp.) cause infected animals to become weak, unthrifty, susceptible to secondary infections, and produce poor quality wool. Lice infestations on chickens (*Liperus caponis*) cause weight loss and reduced egg production.

**FLEAS.** Fleas are much less permanent parasites than lice, frequently leaving their hosts. The dog flea (*Ctenocephalides canis*) and cat flea (*C. felis*) frequently cause human annoyance. The fleas of poultry (*Ceratophyllus gallinae*) and the sticktight flea (*Echidnophoga gallinacea*) may become troublesome in poultry houses. The oriental rat flea (*Xenopsylla cheopsis*) is the principal vector of plague and is not found in the United States; however, other fleas of wild rodents are present and maintain sylvatic plague transmission west of the 100th meridian. Fleas have been incriminated as intermediate hosts of the dog heartworm (*Dirofilaria immitis*) and dog tapeworm (*Dipylidium caninum*).

**MOSQUITOES.** There is a long list of viruses, protozoans, and nematodes that are transmitted to humans and their domestic animals by mosquitoes. The arthropod-borne encephalitides, yellow fever, malaria, and heartworm are only a few, but they illustrate the problem.

### Control

Three approaches to the control of arthropods and arthropod-borne diseases are physical, biological, and chemical. A fourth, integrated pest management, is an increasingly popular concept involving timed utilization of each of the first three methods on a cost-benefit basis. Legal control measures, a fifth form of pest control, can be decreed by federal, state, or local laws and regulations.

**PHYSICAL CONTROL.** The original form of physical control was to physically remove or kill the arthropod pests. In nature it involves grooming among primates; dusting among birds; and biting, rubbing, or scratching among many species of animals. We use it on an individual basis when we detick ourselves or our animals or when we use swatters, adhesive papers, or electrocuters. Physical control may also include measures that restrict or reduce exposure of the host animal to arthropods, such as screening homes and farm buildings.

Other forms of physical control minimize breeding habitats for insect pests. Fly control involves prompt removal and disposal of organic wastes in which fly eggs have been deposited before they undergo larval development and pupation; keeping animal lots or buildings as dry as possible; and removing damp feeds in haystacks, strawpiles, and feed bins. Brush clearing has long been an effective tool in controlling tsetse flies. In Australia an operation known as "mulesing" is performed on sheep to surgically remove the wrinkles from around the anal areas of the animals; this has been a significant advance toward the control of sheep blowfly (*Lucilia cuprina*) for the Australian sheep industry.

Physical control practices are also important for controlling mosquitoes, which can serve as vectors of animal diseases such as Western and Eastern equine encephalitis. Draining lowlands and other types of wet breeding sites by ditching, filling, or removing marginal vegetation from ponds and ditches are examples of physical control measures for mosquito abatement.

**BIOLOGICAL CONTROL.** This type of control usually involves the use of predators, parasites, or pathogens. To date the success of such measures has been rather limited in controlling the insect pests of humans and their domestic animals; however, these techniques have been more widely studied and applied against arthropod pests of plant species.

In addition to using other life forms to attack arthropods, the use of pheromones, growth regulators, irradiation, or chemosterilants can be broadly classified as biological control measures. Pheromones, naturally occurring compounds produced by insects, are used to attract the insects to traps. Growth regulators disrupt growth patterns, interfering with breeding cycles and weather adaptation. Irradiation and chemosterilants have been employed to sterilize mass-reared male insects, which are then released to compete with normal males to reduce or eliminate native insect populations. This technique was the primary tool used in eradicating the screwworm (*Cochliomyia hominivorax*) from the United States.

Breeding tick-resistant cattle and rotating pastures are biological methods of tick control that are used commonly, even without total understanding of the mechanisms of tick resistance. Also, scheduling livestock movements when the vectors are quiescent is another form of biological control.

**CHEMICAL CONTROL.** Insecticides will continue to form the basis for controlling most arthropods during the foreseeable future. Although there are many problems, including possible environmental damage associated with the use of chemicals, to date the advantages have supported their use to the exclusion of most other procedures.

Chemical control includes the following advantages:

1. Insecticides control a wide variety of arthropods. There are those that can control population buildups of ticks, mites, flies, mosquitoes, lice, and other insect pests.

2. There is the possibility of increased productivity. Increased milk production results from stable-fly control, and increased weight gains are achieved

among cattle protected from hordes of mosquitoes. Chemical control of warble flies can prevent hide damage and weight loss in cattle. Dipping to control ectoparasites can improve weight gain.

3. Chemicals can be applied selectively to yield the desired control through a variety of techniques and formulations. They can be effective as sprays, ear tags, collars, dips, feed additives, baits, dust bags, or systemics.

4. Strategic application can be timed to match the life cycle of the parasite or at high-risk periods in the life of the host.

*Modes of Action and Formulations.* Insecticides and pesticides vary widely in the physiological mechanisms by which they alter metabolism in a lethal, behavioral, or developmental manner. Contact poisons kill simply by direct contact, stomach poisons kill when ingested, fumigants are lethal when inhaled, and systemics act after having been taken into the blood of a host animal (without harming the animal host).

Active ingredients are the chemicals in a pesticide product that do the work and can rarely be used in the pure form in which they were made; they usually must be diluted or mixed with something else. Inert ingredients may be added to make the product convenient to handle and safe, easy, and accurate to apply. The mixture of active and inert ingredients is called a formulation. The label directions on the container include precise directions on how to use the formulation, but for proper field use, personnel should be capable of determining concentrations in the final mixture at the site of the dip or spray vat.

Most common types of formulations and their frequently used abbreviations may be referred to in a variety of ways. Liquid formulations include the following:

1. Emulsifiable concentrates (EC) can be mixed directly with water to form emulsions.

2. Solutions (S) are manufactured as high or low concentrates. High concentrates usually contain 8 lb/gal or more of active ingredient, but most are designed to be diluted with oil or petroleum solvents. The low concentrates usually contain less than 2 lb/gal of active ingredient. Many solutions are suitable for livestock sprays and space sprays in barns.

3. Flowables (F or L) have active ingredients that can be made only as a solid, or at best, a semisolid. These are finely ground and put into a liquid with other substances to form a suspension (flowable solids). Flowables can be mixed with water and seldom clog spray nozzles.

4. Aerosols (A) are liquids that contain the active ingredient in solution in a solvent. Most aerosols have a low percentage of active ingredients and are made for use in fog- or mist-generating machines.

5. Gases liquefy when placed under pressure. Liquefied gases usually are

fumigants, stored under either high or low pressure, depending on the material.

Dry formulations include the following:

1. Dusts (D) are ingredients that are ground into fine, uniform particles. The active ingredients usually range from 1 to 10%, with inert ingredients added to improve storage and handling characteristics. Dusts must always be used dry. Some pesticides are available as dust concentrates that must be diluted and mixed with dry inert ingredients before use.

2. Most granular (G) formulations are manufactured by applying a liquid active ingredient to coarse particles (granules) of an inert porous material such as clay, corn cobs, or walnut shells to improve the handling characteristics of the formulation. The active ingredients usually range from 2 to 40%. Granular formulations are safer to apply than ECs or dusts and, like dusts, should always be used dry.

3. Wettable Powders (WP or W) are finely ground pesticide formulations that look like dusts; however, unlike dusts, they are made to mix with water forming a suspension rather than a true solution, so good agitation is needed in the spray tank during their use. Most WPs are much more concentrated than dusts and contain 15–95% active ingredient, usually 50% or more.

4. Soluble Powders (SP) also are dry but, when added to water, form true solutions. Agitation may be needed in the spray tank to get them to dissolve; after that, no more agitation is usually needed. The amount of active ingredient in an SP is usually above 50%.

5. A bait (B) formulation is an edible or attractive substance mixed with a pesticide, which attracts and kills pests after ingestion. The amount of active ingredients in most baits is usually low, less than 5%.

**INTEGRATED CONTROL.** Originally, the term meant the combined use of natural, physical, and chemical procedures to keep pests at tolerable levels. Now the concept usually encompasses all these plus economic-threshold considerations. The terms "threshold population" and "species sanitation" both fit into the integrated-control concept for disease vectors and animal parasites. Threshold population refers to maintaining adequate control to keep general insect population levels below the point at which disease is transmitted at epidemic levels or hosts are parasitized into pathologic conditions. Threshold populations can frequently be attained within a positive cost-benefit basis. Species sanitation refers to directing control measures only against a particular vector or parasite species of importance to health protection. For example, controls are directed only at the principal vector mosquito species (*Culex tarsalis*) of Western encephalitis virus instead of all mosquitoes, or at only the warble fly (*Hypoderma lineatum*) instead of all flies. With the species sanitation concept, the desired control and effects can be attained relatively economically.

**LEGAL CONTROL.** Laws or regulations directed at preventing insect introduction or distribution invoke measures such as quarantines, inspections, and embargoes. There are also laws and regulations directed at labeling, use, and disposal of chemical formulations.

*Regulatory Restrictions.* The Federal Insecticide, Fungicide, and Rodenticide Act (FIFRA) was passed to balance the need for pesticides against the need to protect people and the environment from misuse.

The certification categories most likely applicable to controlling arthropods and vectors of animal diseases by restricted-use pesticides would be agricultural animal pest control, regulatory pest control, or demonstration and research pest control. However, physicians and veterinarians applying pesticides as drugs or medication during the course of their normal practice have been exempted from certification. In most states, certification is administered by a branch of the state government, so those agencies can provide information needed on certification requirements.

Other restrictions involve the shipment of pesticides across state boundaries, which is regulated by the Department of Transportation. Aerial applications of pesticide from aircraft are regulated by the Federal Aviation Administration and also by some state agencies. The Occupational Safety and Health Administration requires anyone with 11 or more workers to keep records and report on work-related pesticide illness, injury, or death under specified circumstances. The Environmental Protection Agency (EPA), under regulations authorized by the Federal Food, Drug, and Cosmetic Act, sets residue tolerances for raw farm products or processed foods.

*Labels.* The pesticide label means many things to different people. To the manufacturer it is documentation of a license to sell the product; to government agencies it provides a method of controlling the distribution, storage, sale, use, and disposal of the material; to the buyer it is a source of facts on how to use the product correctly and legally. It also is a means of advising users about special safety measures needed and may specify when its use (and sale) is restricted to only certified applicators or persons under their direct supervision.

In the United States every pesticide label must list the amount of each active ingredient in the product, given as a percentage by weight or as pounds per gallon of concentrate. The inert ingredients do not have to be named, but the label must show what percent of the total they constitute. The relative toxicity of the product is indicated by signal words: DANGER for highly toxic substances that are fatal to an average person at a dose of no more than a teaspoon, WARNING for moderately toxic substances that are fatal at a dose of a teaspoon to a tablespoon, and CAUTION for substances of low toxicity that are fatal at a dose of an ounce to more than a pint.

The instructions for using the pesticide are an important part of the label and must include the common names of the pests the product is registered to control, the species or target surface it can be used upon, the form in which the pesticide should be applied, how much should be used, where and when it should be applied, and precautionary measures to be followed. Special procedures for avoiding poisoning, such as the need for protective equipment, will be given, and if the product is highly toxic, advice to physicians for the proper treatment for poisoning will be included. Environmental hazards and restrictions, such as avoiding exposure of bees to direct contact or to residues, or avoiding contamination of animal feed, drinking water, milk, and milk-handling equipment, will be listed.

*Problems.* Society's problems associated with using chemicals to control arthropods and arthropod-borne animal diseases include a wide variety of environmental pollution problems, accidental poisonings, and misuses. The relatively uncontrolled use of chemicals, including pesticides, is no longer acceptable to the public in most countries.

Resistance to organic insecticides occurs widely among arthropods, resulting from the survival of some individuals that do not succumb to a particular poison and a natural selection process. Thus, a resistant strain multiplies and replaces the susceptible strains in an insect population. Often, population selection by one type of pesticide hastens the development of resistance against other chemically related compounds that previously were effective. Increasingly restrictive legislation for labeling pesticides, resulting from FIFRA, has greatly increased the costs of developing and marketing new products. Therefore, the number of pesticides now available for use against almost any type of arthropod pest has been drastically reduced.

Disposal of pesticides can also be a problem where large volumes are involved, such as in cattle-dipping vats. Both the pesticide containers and the excess pesticide must be disposed of safely and legally, which includes burning in specially designed pesticide incinerators, burying in specifically designated landfills, or burying in noncroplands away from water supplies. As more has been learned about long-term risk from disposal sites, proper and legal disposition has become more difficult and of greater public concern.

The economics of chemical control are important and should be evaluated on a cost-benefit basis. Chemical control measures generally provide only temporary periods of pest control because they usually do not eliminate the source of the breeding populations; therefore, the expense of periodic retreatments may be considerable. The trend toward limiting the production and sale of long-term residual pesticides also has contributed to the necessity of more frequent retreatments.

# 20

# Cleaning and Disinfection

THE DESIRED END RESULT of cleaning and disinfection procedures in disease control operations is the destruction of pathogens, which cannot be achieved in a one-step application of a disinfectant. These chemicals are effective only upon contact with the pathogens and are ineffective when the pathogens are protected by dirt or tissue, so physical removal of the agent and accompanying soil is essential. (For the purpose of this discussion, the term soil will be used to describe all contaminating material regardless of its physical or chemical characteristics.) After all the material that can be scraped or shoveled away has been removed, cleaning agents can remove the remaining soil.

## Cleaning

The first objective of cleaning is to remove all gross particles of soil to assure a contact between the disinfectant and the pathogens. Despite the inability of most cleaning agents to kill, proper cleaning may physically remove up to 99% of the bacteria from a smooth surface.

Water is the best solvent and cleanser, but its cleaning efficiency is increased greatly by the addition of two broad items: external energy (applied as temperature, time, and force) and cleaning compounds.

An increase in temperature weakens the bond between soil and surface. There is, however, a desired range of temperature. The minimum is 2–3°C above the melting point of the predominant fat in the soil to be removed. Below this minimum, fat removal is difficult. The maximum must be below the denaturation point of the protein present, for if this temperature is exceeded the rate of increase in adhesiveness of denatured protein to the surface is more rapid than the increase in cleaning efficiency.

The optimal time involved in the cleaning operation is important up to a point that must be visually determined. Beyond that point effectiveness decreases. Force is exerted in two forms: the turbulence of the water and the amount of scrubbing pressure or water pressure exerted.

For any cleaning operation to be successful there must be complete access to the item to be cleaned so that ample force and cleaning compound can reach all surfaces. There also must be ample light and visibility to permit visual inspection of the surfaces before, during, and after cleaning. The proper equipment must be in good repair.

Cleaning compounds modify water so it can penetrate, dislodge, and carry away surface contamination. The use of chemical cleaning compounds involves the following steps.

1. Prerinsing minimizes the soil load encountered by the cleaner. Depending on the soil type and the item to be cleaned, up to 90% of the soil can be removed by this step. The optimal water temperature for this operation usually is in the range of 38–46°C.

2. The cleaner should be placed in contact with the soil, usually at a temperature of 49–77°C (some detergents become unstable at higher temperatures). This step requires the cleaning compound to have adequate wetting and penetrating properties.

3. The soil is displaced from the surface. In this operation the fats are saponified, proteins are peptonized, and mineral substances are dissolved.

4. The soil is dispersed in the solvent. Important properties of the cleaning agent in this stage are dispersion, deflocculation, or emulsification.

5. Postrinsing prevents redeposition of the soil on the clean surfaces. To be effective here, the cleaning agent must have good rinsing properties. To prevent suds buildup, it frequently is necessary that the postrinse water be cold, approximately 7–13°C. Timing the postrinse also is important. Although the cleaning agents require time to work, they may be difficult to remove if allowed to remain too long.

In addition to these properties a cleaner should have water softening properties, be quickly and completely dissolved in water, be noncorrosive, nontoxic, economical, stable, and not cake or produce dust in storage and use.

The functions of cleaning agents are sequestering, preventing mineral deposition; wetting, lowering the surface tension of water; emulsifying, fine dispersal of fat and other particles in water; dissolving, speedy transfer of solids into solution; saponifying, turning fats into soap; peptonizing, attaching to and dispersing protein molecules; dispersing, dispersal and flocculation to prevent redeposition; and rinsing, separating freely from the surface with fresh water.

Selection of the proper cleaning compounds requires consideration of the type and amount of soil present (Table 20.1), the nature of the surface (this must be compatible with the cleaning compound to avoid corrosion and staining), the form of the compound to be employed (liquids provide better control of the concentration), and cleaning method to be employed (if hand cleaning is a significant part of the operation, it is essential that the compound be noncorrosive and nonirritating). Also, the availability of the compound and

**Table 20.1.   Cleaning characteristics of various types of soil**

| Soil Type | Solvent | Removal | Changes Under Heat |
|---|---|---|---|
| Sugar | Water | Easy | Caramelization |
| Fat | Alkali | Difficult | Polymerization |
| Protein | Alkali or slight acid | Very difficult | Denaturation |
| Monovalent salt | Water or acid | Easy | Interactions |
| Polyvalent salt | Acid | Difficult | Interactions |

cost per unit surface of the item to be cleaned are important in most operations.

Another important consideration is the water quality, which often is expressed in terms of total solids, i.e., the amount of inorganic salts plus clay, sand, etc. that present serious problems in interaction with cleaning compounds. Hardness, which is reported as grains of calcium carbonate per gallon, is a significant consideration that occurs either as temporary or permanent hardness. Temporary hardness is seen as calcium bicarbonate or magnesium bicarbonate that can be precipitated by heat or chemicals such as sodium hydroxide. Permanent hardness occurs as the sulfates, nitrates, or chlorides of calcium and magnesium and is precipitated by certain alkalies or alkaline salts such as sodium carbonate (soda ash). Both types of hardness cause soap to precipitate and must be removed before permanent suds can be formed.

It is important from a cost standpoint to recognize that cleaning efficiency does not increase at the same rate as the increase of concentration of the compound. An effective and economical way to monitor concentration is by using test kits, often available from the manufacturer.

Although the various classes of cleaning compounds often are combined, they will be discussed as individual items for the sake of simplification. Basically they can be classified as soap, alkalines, amphoteric compounds, acid cleaners, complex phosphates, proteolytic enzymes, surfactants, and chelating agents.

**SOAP.** Soap, the oldest cleaning compound, is a sodium salt of fatty acids formed by the combination of sodium hydroxide (lye) and fat. The interaction with soil is emulsification, where one end of the long organic soap molecule combines in a semipermanent bond with fats and oils and the other end combines with water, permitting the fats and oils to be lifted from the surface. A distinct advantage of soap is its biodegradability; however, it is far less versatile and less effective than most of the newer synthetic compounds.

**ALKALINES.** The basic alkalines displace soil through emulsification, saponification, and peptonization. As a group, they are highly corrosive, good sporicides, and rinse readily, although they do form mineral and protein deposits.

One of the more commonly used basic alkaline cleaners, caustic soda, is highly germicidal and dissolves protein readily but is a poor deflocculant and emulsifier. It also is corrosive to many materials and burns the skin. Soda ash and baking soda are inexpensive and buffer well but are only fair deflocculants and emulsifiers. They function primarily as water softeners.

Trisodiumphosphate (TSP), tetrasodiumphosphate, and sodium hexametaphosphate (quadraphos and calgon) are highly soluble, effective deflocculants and emulsifying agents. They are fair water softeners but are corrosive unless metasilicate has been added as a protective factor. Sodium metasilicate has a high cleaning activity in alkaline solution, is an excellent deflocculant and emulsifier, a water softener, and is relatively noncorrosive compared with other agents in this group.

**AMPHOTERIC COMPOUNDS.** The amphoteric compounds, made of alkylated amino acids such as dodecylbetaalanine, are good wetting agents and emulsifiers and are compatible with anionic, nonionic, and cationic surfactants.

**ACID CLEANERS.** Acid cleaners are most effective as softeners and in removing mineral deposits, and function best at pH 2.5 or less. Most of these acids such as citric, tartaric, or phosphoric, are organic acids of vegetable origin. They are mild, stable, far less corrosive than the alkaline cleaners, can be combined with wetting agents to improve their penetration, and are notable for their ease of rinsing.

**COMPLEX PHOSPHATES.** The complex phosphates are excellent water softeners; good emulsifiers, dispersants, and peptonizers; and prevent redeposition of minerals. The pyrophosphates are the worst in each of the above categories but are the most stable under conditions of high temperature and high alkalinity. Furthermore, they are the cheapest of the phosphates. This entire group serves as nutrients for plant growth, therefore, they create problems as environmental pollutants, which is a distinct disadvantage.

**PROTEOLYTIC ENZYMES.** Proteolytic enzymes are considered classic cleaning compounds but they rarely are used in combination with other compounds. They function only during a presoak.

**SURFACTANTS.** The surfactants (wetting agents) lower the surface tension of water allowing it to penetrate between the soil and the surface to be cleaned. They reduce the attraction between fat molecules and surfaces, acting as penetrating and dispersing agents, thereby preventing redeposition during rinsing. As a group they are soluble in cold water and are relatively unaffected by water hardness, which permits better rinsing in hard water. The large number of categories of surfactants permits selection of an effective agent for water of any pH and any cleaner. With some, even 0.15% will halve the surface tension of water, but there is little value in adding more than this concentration. Surfactants contribute some emulsifying and deflocculating properties but are much less economical in these functions than metasilicates or the phosphate compounds. There are three broad types of surfactants: anionic, nonionic, and cationic. Anionic are most common, work well in hard water, are essentially neutral, and can be used in either acid or alkaline pH, although they function best in alkaline situations. Sulfated alcohols and alkyl aryls, the most common of the anionic group, foam, a characteristic desired by consumers but a problem in sewage disposal systems.

Nonionic surfactants are complex organic compounds that do not ionize, therefore they are compatible with anionic, cationic, and most other cleaners. They usually are acidified to increase their germicidal power.

The best known cationic surfactants, the quaternary compounds, are poor wetting agents, so their greatest use is as germicides or deodorants rather than as cleaners. They operate best in an acid pH.

**CHELATING COMPOUNDS.** Chelating compounds maintain metallic ions in solution, functioning as softeners and controlling mineral deposition. They peptonize to displace the soil, and in precipitate prevention, they function similarly to polyphosphates but are far more heat stable. These compounds are organic acid salts, with each chelater functioning most effectively on a few specific metals, therefore, the cleaning compounds should be tailored for a specific use.

When working with cleaning compounds, safety must be considered. The compounds must be stored and transported in a way that will prevent breakage, spillage, and pilferage, and they must be labeled clearly to avoid confusion with other compounds. During use, protective clothing such as goggles and gloves often is necessary. Workers should be totally familiar with needed concentrations; be qualified to measure and dilute the compounds properly; have the proper equipment readily available for the purpose; and be familiar with any restrictions, special instructions on use, and hazards the compounds may present for animals. Cleaners should be used only where indicated and workers should be schooled in the proper disposal of used and unused material, as well as containers.

If cleaning has been performed properly, no foreign substances will be present to interfere with the action of disinfectants.

## Disinfection

The primary objective of disinfection is to kill pathogens. It is essential that the proper material is selected for each purpose and used in a fresh form at proper concentrations. A 100% kill is seldom possible in a farm situation, and we must be content with reducing the numbers of pathogens below the infecting dose. Since this cannot be measured, it is vital that no shortcuts are taken. Also, it is important to recognize that in addition to killing pathogens, most of these methods involve some hazard for the user as well, requiring protective clothing.

There is a wide diversity in definitions in the field of disinfection, therefore, it is essential to present the definitions as they will be used here.

*Sanitize* — to reduce the numbers of organisms to a relatively safe level. The organisms destroyed are not necessarily pathogens, since sanitizing agents are used where pathogens may not be present or where time or concentrations preclude disinfection. It is a compromise action.

*Disinfect* — to kill most of the vegetative forms of bacteria, fungi, or viruses against which it is directed. For example, a bactericidal disinfectant may be ineffective against fungi. Disinfection does not necessarily mean spores have been killed.

*Sterilize* — to kill all microorganisms present, spores as well as vegetative forms.

*Bacteriostat* — an agent that inhibits multiplication but does not necessarily kill bacteria. Virustatic and fungistatic agents also are available.

*Antiseptic* — an agent that kills or inhibits the growth of micoorganisms, especially on or in living tissues.

*Germicide* — an agent that destroys certain types of microorganisms, e.g., bactericide, fungicide, or virucide. Frequently they are even more specific in their action.

The difference between -static and -cidal agents can be vital in control and eradication efforts: -static agents do not remove pathogens, they merely neutralize them temporarily.

There are three broad approaches to disinfection: heat, radiation, and chemicals.

**HEAT.** Heat is a nonselective killer, functioning essentially by inactivating the protein of the microorganisms. Dry heat accomplishes this through oxidation, moist heat through coagulating the protein. Heat is the only effective approach that eventually will penetrate soil (as earlier defined). Heat dissipates rapidly, which is advantageous from a safety standpoint but is a serious problem if not applied long enough to destroy the pathogens. However, heat has no residual action and is often inconvenient to use. It is the safest approach because the hazard usually is readily apparent.

**RADIATION.** Radiation penetrates poorly, is poor at destroying spores, has no residual action, usually is inconvenient, and requires elaborate safety precautions. Because of public awareness today, use of radiation would probably create greater public antagonism toward the program.

**CHEMICALS.** Chemical disinfection is convenient in that most chemicals are relatively portable, but the concentration must be checked periodically to assure effective and safe operation. In the United States all chemical disinfectants are registered with the Environmental Protection Agency. An evaluation technique established by the Association of Official Analytical Chemists consists of preparing a dried film of the test organism, exposing it to the test chemical in the recommended dilution, then transferring the cylinder to a broth in which it is incubated. The phenol coefficient is a common measure but it provides sufficient evaluative information only against *Salmonella typhi* and *Staphylococcus aureus* and should not be used in evaluation agents to be employed against other pathogens.

Because of the selective nature of most chemical disinfectants, the USDA has established a list of recommended chemicals for use against certain animal pathogens; the listing is maintained by the Emergency Field Operations staff, Veterinary Services, APHIS, USDA.

There are many commonly used sanitizers or disinfectants.

Alcohols, in the ethyl and isopropyl form, are most effective in 60–95% dilutions. Methyl alcohol is toxic and a poor bactericidal agent. Alcohols are excellent solvents but are highly flammable.

Glycols are used essentially as aerosols or mists and have relatively limited utilization.

Formaldehyde usually is used as a gaseous sporicide and disinfectant. It requires at least 70% humidity and penetrates poorly. Gluteraldehyde has some medical uses.

Ethlyene oxide is a gas with some flaming and explosive tendencies. The equipment and control measures necessary for its use are detractions.

Heavy metals such as mercury and arsenic have relatively limited usefulness because of their high toxicity.

Acid sanitizers usually are a combination of acid plus anionic surfactants. Although slow acting, they are stable, nonselective killers that denature cellular proteins and increase cell wall permeability. They function best in a pH of 1.9–2.2, are nonstaining, and are odorless, although they often produce a foam.

The phenolic compounds denature proteins by entering the cell and combining with proteins at the sites with positive charges. The proteins then are unable to function effectively. Phenolics are insoluble in water, have strong odors, and are easily inactivated by proteins and soaps but not by hard water. They are highly alkaline, functioning best at their use concentration at a pH of approximately 10.

The quaternary compounds denature intracellular enzymes and also directly attack the cell wall, which increases its permeability and produces cytoplasmic leakage. The positively charged end of the quaternary compound combines with negative sites on the cell wall, eventually causing the membrane to cease functioning and break apart. These compounds are slow acting and until the wall has totally broken apart, the inactivation can be reversed by negatively charged long-chain molecules. After use, they should be rinsed to avoid deactivation by soap. This group of compounds is relatively selective in that they are inactive against the *Mycobacteria,* most of the viruses, and most of the gram-negative organisms, especially *Pseudomonas.* They have some detergent properties but usually are formulated with nonionic detergents added, decreasing the kill rate. They are mild, noncorrosive, nontoxic, leave a residual bacteriostatic film, prevent odors, penetrate well, and are stable to heat, pH, and most organic compounds. They are not compatible with phosphates, soaps, proteins, or anionic detergents; are expensive; slow acting; foam readily; and are effective in neutral to alkaline solutions in the pH range 7–10.

The halogens, chlorine and iodine, kill by oxidizing at sites with nitrogen, sulfur, or carbon ions. They also have significant bleaching properties in addition to their sanitizing abilities.

Chlorine usually is employed as a hypochlorite. The sodium form is unstable as a powder, therefore it usually is supplied as a liquid. Calcium chloride forms precipitate and scale with some organic material and releases a gas at a pH less than 5, with its primary activity due to formation of hypochlorous acid. The hypochlorites are cheap and quick, nonselective killers, effective sporicides, readily soluble, and operate effectively in hard water, although an iron concentration of greater than 1 ppm will produce a precipitate, rendering the chlorine inactive. They are easily measured, dispensed, and their concentrations controlled, but they have a relatively short shelf life, are corrosive, and dissipate readily in use. The active form, hypochlorous acid, oxidizes the essential enzymes of cells, thereby disrupting metabolism. Secondarily, it reacts with proteins in the cell membrane and cytoplasm, yielding toxic nitrogenous chlorocompounds. Unfortunately, any protein compounds in the water will react with the chlorine to form chloramines that are relatively slow acting, and chlorines deteriorate quickly in the presence of organic matter.

Iodine is a very effective, nonselective disinfectant that forms protein salts and destroys cellular enzymes. However, because of its corrosive nature it usually is combined with a nonionic surfactant to produce iodophores, which have a long shelf life; are fast acting, nonselective killers; are noncorrosive; are easily dispensed and measured; work well in hard water; have good penetrating power; and prevent film and spot formation. They also are expensive, inoperative over 49°C, only fair sporicides, require a low pH (less than 7 and preferably in the 3–4 range), and stain plastics. Because of their mild nature, they can be used on the hands with no problems, and have the distinct advantage of a color indicator showing when they are effective. This amber color is present down to 6–8 ppm in water, yet 5 ppm will kill 99.99% of any vegetative bacterial cells within 30 seconds of contact, if the surface is clean. In hard or dirty water, 25 ppm of iodine is the equivalent of 100 ppm chlorine. Up to 10 ppm iodophores will not produce a flavor in milk. The iodophores are fairly effective in the presence of organic matter, but they will not dissolve protein as effectively as the alkaline detergents.

In the presence of organic matter, quaternary compounds are most effective with iodophores next, followed by hypochlorites, the least effective. The pH is another important consideration in choice of disinfectants. The germicidal activity is increased with high pH in the quaternary compounds and with low pH with chlorine. Iodine is less sensitive but most effective at lower pHs.

## Evaluation

One of the unresolved problems associated with soil removal and pathogen destruction is how to determine the adequacy of the procedure. Cleaning is usually evaluated by visual inspection with the results subjectively compared with the evaluator's concept of what is satisfactory. For disinfection there are more objective but oblique methods: test strips for autoclaves, phosphatase tests for pasteurization, bacteriologic quantitation after water purification, various colorimetric tests for determining disinfectant concentrations. The fact remains, however, that the only valid method available today for field evaluation of cleanup and disinfection procedures is the costly and time-consuming use of sentinel animals. This lack of quick, easy evaluation techniques places a grave responsibility on the individual who plans, supervises, and approves these operations.

# 21

# Disposal and Indemnity

COMPULSORY DISPOSAL of infected or exposed animals as an element of disease control or eradication is routinely applicable only to controlled (domesticated) populations. Wild populations, even if important in the epidemiology of a disease, usually are not amenable to reduction to a level that would significantly reduce the rate of pathogen transmission. For that reason, advance consideration of the role of wildlife (Chap. 17) is essential when developing plans for control or eradication of a pathogen.

In most countries, utilizing compulsory disposal as part of an animal health program also includes a system of indemnification for the affected owners. This is important, not only for reasons of equity, but also to maintain owner cooperation.

Although controlled slaughter is one of the most important disease eradication tools in countries where the economic and ethical climate permits its use, it is a complex subject with technical, political, financial, and social ramifications. Unfortunately, this importance is seldom matched by equivalent attention to prior training of health personnel and study of techniques for field application. Deliberate destruction is not an inviting endeavor for those whose profession is prevention of disease and preservation of life, neither is it pleasant for the owners who have devoted their life to breeding and raising livestock. Slaughter is only valid when it is essential to prevent further spread of infection into the susceptible population. If slaughter will not accomplish this purpose it has no place in the program.

Organized government effort is required to effectively employ a national or regional slaughter policy. In 1870, when foot-and-mouth disease virus entered the United States for the first time, there was no established regulatory mechanism, no slaughter policy. By 1884, with the creation of the United States Bureau of Animal Industry, it was possible to include systematic disposal in the country's first disease eradication program, directed against contagious bovine pleuropneumonia.

Among the decisions to be made in structuring an eradication program are whether or not slaughter must be used, at what stage to start slaughter if it is necessary, what categories of animals or herds should be included, and when to stop. These decisions depend largely on adequate prior knowledge of the cycle and prevalence of the disease. If slaughter is started without this knowledge, it may fail to meet its part of the program mission.

Once a decision is made that a slaughter policy is needed, additional questions arise. From a technical standpoint these include not only the extent and method of the slaughter process but also disposition of the carcasses, environmental impact concerns, cleaning and disinfection of the premises involved, how long such premises should be vacated, and how such premises should be restocked. Beyond these technical points it is essential to consider the economic, social, political, and animal welfare aspects of slaughter. Each of these needs to be studied in relation to the particular situation involved.

## Slaughter

Slaughter can range from a single infected animal to all susceptible animals in a given area. Slaughter of a single infected animal is one way to get started against an established disease that spreads relatively slowly; this can produce progress relatively inexpensively for a considerable time and has frequently been done with bovine tuberculosis and brucellosis. Even with brucellosis and tuberculosis, however, there eventually will be situations where it is necessary to remove exposed animals and infected herds.

The other extreme, while drastic, appears at first glance to be uncomplicated in administration and effective in result. In actuality, widespread total elimination of animals poses large political, economic, and technical questions. Destruction of an entire species in an area of any size is costly and causes antagonism among the people in the region. Technically, it is hard to know how widespread the exposure has been and consequently how large the area of destruction should be. However, it is possible to use this technique on a large scale, as demonstrated in recent years in Malta, the Dominican Republic, and Haiti, where the entire swine population was eliminated following the introduction of African swine fever virus.

In most circumstances, an efficient system to promptly locate and eliminate infected and exposed herds or flocks is an effective parameter for a slaughter policy. Exposure usually has occurred by proximity of residence or by additions; the emphasis should be on the herd, not the animal. Few agents against which a slaughter policy is mounted can be restricted effectively by removing only the infected animals. If slaughter is limited to this category, the program constantly will be trying to catch up with spread of infection rather than getting ahead of the problem.

In estimating the necessary extent of slaughter, which usually means defining the extent of exposure, the emphasis should be on eradication, particularly in the latter stages of a program when hesitancy to destroy animals delays, and possibly endangers, final eradication.

**METHODS.** Slaughter techniques in disease eradication programs have ranged from sending condemned animals to the slaughterhouse to destroying them by gunfire, captive-bolt firearms, lethal gases, and injection of lethal drugs. None are pleasant on a farm or ranch, especially when dealing with large numbers of animals. The physical arrangements available and the experience of those doing the work are seldom comparable to the facilities and experience at a slaughterhouse, which is organized for efficient, rapid destruction. However, when slaughterhouses are used extreme care must be taken to assure that the pathogen does not find its way back into the livestock population via plant employees, waste products, and the products themselves.

In many countries there is increased public concern over humane treatment of animals. In the United States these concerns have resulted in national legislation, from the Humane Slaughter Act of 1958 to the more recent Animal Welfare and Horse Protection acts. Program slaughter methods have been, and will continue to be, affected by these increased sensitivities. The American Veterinary Medical Association (AVMA) has studied methods of euthanasia, including those used in regulatory programs, and has raised questions about some procedures (AVMA 1978, 1986).

Both professional standards and public attitudes emphasize a need to cease thinking of slaughter methods in programs requiring animal disposal and think instead in terms of systems for euthanasia, which has been defined as painless, peaceful death. With this definition our approach to improved techniques starts from a base appropriate to modern demands.

Dr. J. E. Braezile defined the ideal destruction system in eradication programs as being humane, safe for the applicant, easy to use, and inexpensive. It also should be rapid, reliable, esthetically satisfactory for observers and operator and interrupt consciousness and reflex mechanisms simultaneously. It is difficult to find a single agent that meets all these requirements; increased study in recent years includes emphasis on the humane aspects of the systems reviewed.

Improved techniques are needed, but the most important element is the experience and sensitivity of the person in charge, particularly when a large number of animals are to be destroyed in the field. It is an important, yet unpleasant, responsibility that requires prior training, meticulous preplanning, good organization, and concern for the condemned animals as well as the feelings of the owners and others involved.

**DISPOSAL.** Disposal of carcasses has been by commercial slaughter, rendering, burning, or burial. Commercial slaughter or rendering is efficient for relatively small numbers, if facilities can be found in the area that will accept the animals and if it is economically efficient to provide safeguards against agent spread. Obviously, these methods should not be considered if the end products cannot be made safe.

In recent years, perhaps due to heightened public concern regarding food quality and safety, many slaughterers have been reluctant to handle such animals. Because of animal health risk, concern over human exposure to disease, and meat inspection requirements, regulatory restrictions often reduce prices paid for salvaged animals sent to slaughter.

During the U.S. eradication program against vesicular exanthema of swine (1952–1956), many herds were sent to slaughter, with the meat subjected to sterilization through special heat processing. The prices paid were generally low in comparison to the prevailing market price. When the hog cholera eradication program started in 1962, the meat industry was reluctant to specially process swine, thus the procedure was not used.

Efficient burning or burial requires experience and organization. Burning demands large volumes of fuel, for the carcasses alone will not sustain combustion. Adding carcasses to a burning pyre demands caution if it is not in an incinerator designed for that purpose, and there is likely to be an air pollution problem.

Burial can only be accomplished if ample space and excavation equipment are available. (In nations with a surplus of labor it may be advisable to dig the pit manually.) Points to consider for the selection of a burial site are (1) topography and soil profile, (2) possible pollution of ground water (consult with civil engineers), and (3) accessibility for carcass transport. If burial is to be used, the carcasses should be slashed before they are covered to permit gas to escape as they decay. Many of these technical matters result from the high level of public concern over environmental protection. Even if the agencies responsible for administering environmental legislation are satisfied with disposal arrangements, local groups may not agree and may intervene.

All these difficulties do not mean that traditional means of carcass disposal can no longer be used. However, they do mean that thorough preplanning for probable contingencies, with the various interest groups arriving at a mutually acceptable solution, is necessary to reduce risk of delay in carrying out field programs.

**HANDLING OF PREMISES.** After the condemned animals are removed, the premises require attention. The two questions that generally arise are (1) how long should the property be vacant and (2) are controls needed over the numbers and susceptibility of animals used for restocking? These will vary with the disease.

Following cleaning and disinfection (Chap. 19) a decision is needed on how long to hold the premises free of susceptible animals; a vacation period is an added insurance factor. The length of time will depend on the ability of the agent to survive outside the body, the physical characteristics of the premises, and the local climate. Climate must be considered for there is a marked difference in potential risk between a facility vacated for 30 days in the heat of summer and one vacated for 30 days in subfreezing winter temperatures. Any decision to keep premises vacant, and for how long, should be based on valid technical reasons applying to the situation and the aims of the program. It should not be based on a vague assumption that it might be "a good thing to do." A vacancy period is a further economic burden on the owner, and government authority is abused if it is exercised without specific need. Idle pastures and facilities produce no income, but fixed costs such as maintenance and taxes continue.

The restocking policy also will depend on the situation. For a disease for which there is field program experience, thorough cleaning and disinfection followed, if necessary, by a scientifically supportable vacation period should be sufficient to protect the owner's investment in replacement animals. For a unique situation such as a primary outbreak of a previously exotic disease, public financing for limited restocking with animals of known susceptibility is desirable.

The proper handling of premises requires careful analysis during program planning and should be modified if program experience dictates. It should not be handled superficially, i.e., treated as something required by regulations but not really too important. Nothing should be required that is not necessary, but the actions that are necessary should be followed strictly. It is not pleasant for the owner or program personnel to have a new herd become infected after the premises have been released as being free of residual infection.

**ECONOMIC CONSIDERATIONS.** Direct costs of a slaughter program are costs to the public for indemnities, disposal, and cleaning and disinfection. To these are added owner costs to the extent that indemnities do not cover the value of animals or materials destroyed and that vacation time of the premises is uncompensated. Direct costs can be estimated with more confidence than indirect costs.

Market disruptions can have a marked impact on a variety of economic levels in an area heavily affected by a stamping-out program. For example, when the egg producers in southern California were hit hard by the Newcastle disease virus eradication program in the early 1970s, a whole complex of businesses dependent on the poultry industry was affected: haulers, processors, feed dealers, hatcheries, and even corner lunchrooms near the egg plants. These costs could not be measured accurately, but locally they were perceived to be large enough to provoke demands to stop the program. Since the affected area was localized these demands did not stop the program. A different scale of complaint would have resulted if there had been a large-scale slaughter effort involving livestock over wide areas of the country: livestock markets could be closed; the meat supply chain interrupted; and public reaction to mounting direct and indirect costs, coupled with market disruption, could endanger continuation of the program. That is why the initial attack on a newly introduced, potentially destructive disease needs to be an all-out affair. It is the optimum time to do what is needed and may be the only time at which it can be done.

Direct costs are the costs program administrators find of greatest concern, frequently due to indemnity costs rising to the point that continued funding is questioned. One way to reduce direct costs is to salvage indemnified animals for food. In the United States reactors to brucellosis or tuberculosis testing have been salvaged for many years by being sent to slaughter under specific controls. For several years during the U.S. hog cholera eradication program, apparently healthy swine from infected herds were salvaged to stretch indemnity funds as a trade-off, for some risk to the program was involved. The procedure was halted when the program reached a point where the risk of spreading infection exceeded savings in indemnities. A similar practice existed at one time in the program against scrapie in sheep, but it stopped when research results raised the question of possible risk to human health.

Two studies in the 1970s on the economic value of animal protein conservation were made in connection with contingency planning regarding foot-and-mouth disease (FMD). A work group convened by the animal health agency of the United States Department of Agriculture (USDA) recommended a formula for estimating value (USDA 1973). The price received for the salvaged animal is added to the saved (avoided) cost of disposal if the animal was disposed of on the farm; the cost of maintenance and transportation prior to slaughter is subtracted from this total. If the result is greater than zero, salvage pays for itself.

The second study (Aulaqi 1979) concerned the potential economic impact of FMD in the United States. Part of the report was an estimate of the costs of carcass disposition. Using the estimates from these reports, with some assumptions of possible salvage prices, it is possible to estimate what salvage might save in terms of net value. The cheapest carcass disposal cost (an estimated $0.57 per carcass) occurred when carcasses were buried using large bulldozers. Packers seldom pay market price for salvaged animals, so with an estimated packer price at 50% of the general market value, a 1000-lb cow in a $6.00/cwt market would return $300.00. The total salvage price and cost saved by avoiding burial would be $300.57. If it cost less than $300.57 to maintain the condemned cow and move it to slaughter, then salvage would pay off in program savings, not including value to the consumer from added protein in the food chain.

This is neat and orderly, and probably unrealistic, for it assumes availability of processing plants with the desire and capacity to properly handle the carcasses. The work group that studied animal protein conservation concluded that these plants did not exist in sufficient volume in the United States in 1973 for salvage in an FMD program. The system also assumes that salvage can be carried out safely as far as disease eradication is concerned and that the public would be willing to allow animals under restriction to enter the food supply.

While direct economic impact of a slaughter program can be estimated in some detail, other factors, including willingness of packers and the public to allow salvage procedures, can be expected to have more influence on what is done than purely economic considerations. This is particularly applicable to large salvage programs.

## Indemnities

When property is condemned for the public good, indemnities are necessary in most countries having an economic system based on private ownership. In the United States national animal disease eradication programs requiring condemnation of privately owned animals have always included payment of indemnities. In most instances payment has been shared between national and state governments.

Indemnity payments commonly have been based on the market value of the condemned animal or product at the time of appraisal; a relatively simple method applied effectively when there is a current, accepted market for the type, class, or grade of the animal or product being appraised. It is more difficult to establish an appraisal price for breeding stock or producing animals such as milk cows or laying hens, for the anticipated future return may not be reflected in any current market price structure. It has been argued that an appraisal system based on estimated future productivity is more equitable. In the Newcastle disease eradication program in California, laying hens were appraised on a sliding scale by age, with potential based on the producer's production history and income determined by egg prices in local markets (USDA 1978). Such a system, based on productivity, evolved as the basis of calculating indemnities shifted from current market value to one based on computing (subsequent to slaughter) the estimated value of future productivity. The assistance of an economist is essential if such a system is to function properly.

The advantages and disadvantages of both approaches were identified by Aulaqi and Sundquist (1979) (Table 21.1). The market value appraisal system can be complicated in large programs. The estimated future productivity system is much more complex and should be used only in instances where no other approach will accomplish the purpose, if used at all. The complexity arises from predictions that must be made of production levels, length of productive life, and future market values.

In addition to a clear, general concept of indemnification as a tool for disease control or eradication, program personnel should be well versed in the indemnity regulations applicable to the programs with which they work. In developing an understanding of the use of indemnities in disease programs, there are some factors to keep in mind.

1. The primary purpose of indemnity is to benefit the public by eliminat-

**Table 21.1. Advantages and disadvantages of indemnities based on the current market value and future productivity**

| Advantages | Disadvantages |
|---|---|
| *Current Market Value* | |
| Simple, impersonal, easily administered | Temporary gains or losses due to market fluctuation |
| Requires little time and personnel cost | Market prices not available if markets are closed in outbreak areas |
| Adjustable for quantitive, qualitative, seasonal, and locational differences | Does not account specifically for "lost income" (future productivity) |
| *Future Productivity* | |
| Can incorporate downtime or secondary income losses | Costly in time and personnel |
| Particularly appropriate where future breeding or productivity value is of great importance | Must be based on estimates of the future, can be grossly inaccurate |
| | Difficult to maintain equitability between efficient and inefficient producers |

ing sources for further spread of disease, not to compensate owners. Indemnity funds are appropriated for public benefit, not for individual disaster relief.

2. Constant attention must be given to maintaining an equitable balance between the owner wanting to get as much as he can and the government wanting to pay as little as possible. Payments that are too low reduce owner cooperation and may result in an unwillingness to report suspicious illness. Payments that are too high may promote artificially induced infection; they also divert funds away from other parts of the program or other needs of society.

3. Expert appraisers should be a part of every large slaughter program. In practice, such experts may not always be available, making it prudent that staff analysis and procedural development are carried out prior to and during a program. Routine field appraisals will be done by program staff who are not, by training, professional marketing people; training in appraisal for those who will be called upon to do it will benefit the program, the public, and the appraisers themselves.

4. Industry confidence in the fairness of the indemnity system is important to program success. Confidence requires understanding, which in turn requires sound public information efforts, during the program as well as preceding it.

5. Payment should be prompt. Nothing irritates owners more than finding, after the stresses of condemnation and disposal of their herds, that they have to confront a series of bureaucratic layers with a business-as-usual attitude. Few regulatory procedures are effective if they are performed at a leisurely pace and this includes the administration of indemnity payments. Further, if payment is delayed, the operator may face real cash-flow problems

in operations such as dairies and laying houses where a regular cash flow is needed.

## Sociopolitical Factors

The factors just discussed plus the need for slaughter, the humaneness of the procedures employed, the sensitivity of program officials, the cost in terms of public funds, waste of animal protein, and the risk to human health are all influenced by public perception. These are particularly evident in programs with a high level of slaughter over widespread geographic areas.

The human health factor can involve both the disease that is targeted by the program and an environmental concern over the impact of program procedures. The disease risk factor is illustrated in changing attitudes toward the handling of bovine brucellosis reactors in the United States, where for many years such reactors have been sent for regular slaughter. A public interest group expressed concern over a possible public health threat through salvaging these brucellosis reactors. The National Brucellosis Technical Commission (1978b) stated that occupational health standards for handling reactor cattle may eventually be imposed on the meat industry unless the hazard to packing-plant personnel is reduced. The report also pointed out that two states then restricted entry of brucellosis reactors for slaughter and that other states were investigating reports of brucellosis in packinghouse employees. A far greater problem would arise if the meat from these reactors was viewed by consumers as a potential health hazard.

Environmental concerns have required adjustment of on-site disposal procedures for those occasions when large animals are slaughtered. The public is increasingly conscious of such items as contamination of ground water supplies. Concern over air quality will inhibit the latitude for open-air burning of large numbers of carcasses, although this method, if properly done, is so expensive compared with burial that it would be difficult to justify except in unusual situations. This means that selected burial sites, approved by environmental control agencies, may be needed in any large program. Even then local protest groups may object and court actions may result, regardless of official approval. Those involved in disposal of large numbers of chemically contaminated carcasses have already experienced this type of problem.

As mentioned earlier, there is heightened public interest in humane treatment of animals. This concern has applications to the conduct of slaughter programs and goes beyond the need for improved methods for euthanasia. Monitoring by animal welfare groups is always a possibility, but monitoring by the press is a certainty in any large effort. Time spent explaining what is to be done, and why, may not always produce understanding. However, if the effort is not made, the resulting publicity can be expected to emphasize the sensational rather than the informational.

One point often missed in discussing animal health programs is the reduction of suffering in the general population through eliminating disease. While the primary purpose for most programs is economic, it is entirely proper to discuss the humanitarian aspects of a successful effort. For example, little publicity has been directed toward the relief that wild animals have experienced as a result of screwworm eradication in the United States. Successful eradication efforts, whether of human or other animal pathogens, is an investment in the health and well-being of future generations.

Therefore, technical correctness is not enough. Sensitivity toward the people and livestock involved is an additional responsibility of the field supervisor. If parts of the program are perceived to be improper, the large public benefits of the program may be lost. Anyone who has dealt with newspeople during a dramatic field program that includes on-site slaughter knows that the first thing reporters and photographers want is access to the slaughter process. This kind of interest cannot be avoided and any attempt to do so is liable to produce accusations of cover-up. It is important to work in a way that can be justified in terms of social standards.

A related subject, as far as public sensitivity is concerned, is reactions to a stamping-out program that includes reduction of susceptible wildlife by slaughter. Opposition can be expected from private sources and, if there is no advance discussion, from wildlife management agencies.

Although the purpose of a slaughter program is clear, the execution of that policy requires detailed planning and execution if the work is to be done properly. To expect field personnel to learn by doing is to assume this activity is unimportant. There is nothing simple about the proper disposition of condemned herds and flocks in either large-scale emergency programs or less dramatic long-term programs. Planning and training for this facet of a program, including hands-on experience, is as important as training for diagnosis and epidemiology.

# 22

# Financial and Legal Aspects

ANIMAL HEALTH PROGRAMS require specialized scientific and technical expertise and are usually directed by professionals whose academic training did not include business or management subjects. Yet the program director, usually a veterinarian, has responsibility for all, including nonmedical functions.

It is not unusual for those with a science background to approach program management with a belief that the nonscientific functions can be left to the business or administrative staff and the legal advisors in order to save valuable time. While the program director, presumably placed in that position because of professional expertise and leadership qualities, should not try to become expert in all details of all support functions, the financial and legal aspects of the work are two functions that are critical for comprehensive program management.

A truism of the exercise of authority is that those who control the funds control the operation. A program director who lets others manage the money will eventually lose actual control of the work. For government programs, operation on a sound footing requires legal authority to proceed; additions or changes must similarly be founded on authority to act. Program progress requires the leadership to be conversant with these authorities.

Neither of these areas may be appealing to one trained in another professional field, but organizational leadership usually means that a large block of time must be spent in areas not specifically related to early academic background. Complex programs include a variety of functions beyond the technical and scientific basis of the work. The program leader is the one individual who must have an overview of the total effort to keep all the elements working together. The effective leader is a generalist, not a specialist, and must be able to handle many different aspects in knowledgeable fashion.

### Finances

Funding is the fuel of a program but is seldom available in the amount desired. The program leader must decide how the available funds will be used for the best overall results. This requires more than the ability to read a balance sheet. A thorough understanding of the budget process, how funds are finally obtained, the restrictions placed on how funds can be spent, and the control process for such expenditures is necessary.

**BUDGET.** The key management tool for nonemergency programs, starting with initial planning and continuing throughout the campaign, is the program budget. Everything should come together during budget development: essential elements of the program must be identified, costs of each activity must be estimated, and each required category needs justification that will withstand challenge. This justification covers the technical feasibility of the action, why it is necessary in this particular program, and why the funding level requested is required.

Proposed budgets are normally subject to review at several levels: the parent agency, the department, the central budget office, and if it survives these hurdles, the legislative bodies that recommend funding. Planners at each of these levels should critically review all the categories and justifications that comprise the total.

Health programs usually require expertise that is outside the experience of those who will pass judgment on the budget, and health program leadership must guard against leaving an impression that, as the resident experts, they are present to instruct the uninformed in what must be done rather than to explain why they believe it should be done. An attitude that the amount requested is nonnegotiable, and that if the full amount is not received dire consequences will follow, is a sure way to arouse resentment and increase the probability of an adverse decision.

The granting authorities may not fully appreciate the technology required for the program, but they do understand the budget process and the reality of competition for funding, and effective leadership includes being able to argue the case within that framework.

However, a budget presentation in an emergency situation is made in an atmosphere of urgency, and there is seldom any need to argue that something must be done. The pressures on the program agency are not for justifications for action but for rapid and effective results. In fact, if the public is aroused and apprehensive, which is often the case, political levels may urge unnecessary actions that would be a diversion of manpower, perhaps beyond the technical capability of any operating agency.

In this instance program leaders must be cautious about accepting funding for activities that are unnecessary or cannot be achieved. Postprogram audits, done after the furor has died down, are not inclined to be charitable toward unneeded expenses or activities identified but not accomplished.

Budget requests for either emergency or nonemergency programs call for as much realism as is possible within the time frame permitted and the depth of knowledge then available. Beyond this the aim in nonemergency requests is to create understanding and agreement that the work is needed for the public benefit; in emergency situations the program agency may need to dampen unrealistic assumptions that the application of money will be equivalent to efficiency and results.

It is axiomatic that funds actually received will usually vary, generally downward, from the amount initially requested; a revised financial plan is then required. The program director must decide whether the original time schedule can still be met, whether some elements of the program can be postponed or eliminated, and how the funds finally granted should be allocated to best accomplish program objectives.

These decisions require judgment beyond simply applying an across-the-board percentage cut, a method frequently applied by political levels confronted with need for broad reductions, for technical judgments are not required and complaints of interest groups are reduced. Instead, effective use of the amounts finally appropriated requires selective judgment based on what will have the least effect on the total program. The director is in the best position to evaluate the total program, and the director should make the final decisions on the allocation of funds. Effective exercise of this responsibility requires the director to have confidence in dealing with finances and experience in judging the effects of fund changes on program activities. Finance officers or technical staff should not be expected to exercise this responsibility.

**FINANCIAL CONTROL.** Financial control goes beyond the periodic distribution by the finance officer of account sheets that compare allocations with expenditures. A necessary first step is to learn how to interpret the accounting sheets, as is the necessity for learning how to read a map before trying to use it in the field.

Financial control of a program is more than looking at the totals to see if they are a plus or a minus. Predicting trends from financial records is an important part of program operation that requires not only familiarity with the numbers, but periodic briefing and critiques involving line leadership, financial officers, and program staff. These sessions are particularly important toward the end of the spending cycle so that unpleasant financial surprises can be avoided. It is poor program management to unexpectedly run out of money before the end of the fiscal year or, even worse, find that overspending has already taken place. Such events slow or stop program activity and undermine confidence in the management capabilities of the operating agency.

Cost projections for indemnity expenses are particularly difficult; exact predictions of the number of infected or exposed animals or herds is not really possible, particularly as a program reaches full operating levels.

In some countries where indemnity costs are drawn from the general treasury as needed and are not part of the operating appropriations, this is not a problem unless the cost gets so high that the whole program is threatened. In the United States indemnity costs for nonemergency programs must be estimated in advance and are appropriated in a specific amount as part of the operational funds. Financial analysis and frequent cost projections are particularly important to prevent fund shortages at a time that may be critical for program momentum.

Constant awareness of how actual expenditures compare with the program plan is one of the responsibilities of the program director.

## Legal Foundations

Public programs are conducted under legal authority delegated by the appropriate governing level. The program director must thoroughly understand that authority and its limitation. The authority to act cannot be assumed in structuring a new program or in altering the course of one already underway.

The same applies to the field staff, who must have a general knowledge of basic program authorities and a good knowledge of the regulations drawn under those authorities. Field professionals should be informed of the legal base for their actions and how far that base extends.

In the United States where most animal health programs are operated under both state and federal authority, it is essential that both parties know they have authority to do what is required of them: Is there authority to require reporting of suspicion of the disease in question, to order forced disposal of exposed or infected animals or herds, to ban sales or movement of designated classes of animals or designated animal products?

Correction of potential legal problems before a program starts is obviously preferable to confronting those problems after the program is underway. It is not uncommon, for example, to find that authorities used to act successfully against one disease are not automatically transferable to a program against another disease.

Prudent planning and direction require program leaders to seek sound legal advice before proceeding in any area for which this has not been done. They may elect not to follow that advice if they feel that there are overriding reasons to do so, but obtaining legal counsel is an important part of the decision-making process.

A situation that frequently confronts a program director is how to find a route of action through what seems to be a wall of legal complications brought up by legal advisors. However, this problem may be more apparent than real.

It is not the function of legal counsel to rubber stamp every proposed action. The counsel's first task is to search for all possible legal pitfalls and point them out. Experienced program leaders will further review their aims with the legal staff to find a way that is legally supportable and will still accomplish the desired result.

For most operating programs, regulations drawn under applicable laws constitute the working foundation for program procedures; regulatory personnel deal with regulations every day and with basic law infrequently.

In the United States both federal and state animal health regulations usually originate in the program agency, subject to legal review for correct terminology and structure. Therefore, as an experienced counsel for the USDA once observed, most of the difficulties program agencies have with the regulations under which they operate are problems the agency creates for itself by focusing too narrowly on the one thing they want to achieve and failing to foresee larger complications they may be creating. Therefore, the task of preparing program regulations requires the ability to look beyond the immediate objective. A major weakness in any regulation, other than obscure language, a bureaucratic tendency that must be constantly fought, is trying to cover every contingency with such specific requirements that no latitude is provided for meeting unforeseen circumstances.

Adoption of poorly drawn regulations leads to unwieldy or unworkable sections that cannot be uniformly enforced. Correction is time consuming and an admission of earlier poor judgment; these may accumulate to a point where the agency informally operates under an unwritten policy of selective enforcement (selecting specific occasions to apply the requirements and ignoring others). This pitfall, which most regulatory agencies fall into at one time or another, is not only poor legal practice but also reduces public confidence in the work of the agency. It also has a damaging effect on the attitude of field personnel when they realize that the regulations are not always enforced as written.

An additional pitfall may arise when an operating agreement for an international program is being drawn. The director of the program agency may be careful to draft language stipulations that will provide some limits on the costs or responsibilities of the country. Most such agreements circulate upward in draft form before final signing, and the original draft leaves the program agency subject to alteration. If the program agency loses touch with the draft and subsequent alterations are made, the final product may emerge in changed form. Once signed, the part becomes legally binding, even if the meaning in the original draft has been changed.

An example based on an experience in U.S. animal health work involved a draft proposal prepared by an experienced program advisor: military surplus vehicles would be supplied to carry out certain field activities in an international campaign. As the original draft language moved up in the clearance process, the words "military surplus" were deleted so that the final agreement said only that vehicles would be provided. The final agreement, with the altered wording, became legally binding, and it was necessary for the United States to furnish all vehicles.

As with budgeting and financial control, legal foundations for program work are such an integral part of program leadership that those in this position must make this portion of the work a part of their activity.

# 23

# Audits and Investigations

THERE IS A FOLK STORY, found in many cultures, of the prince, surrounded by courtiers in the palace, who disguises himself in beggar's garments and slips into the countryside to inspect the real world. In modern times we have a structured system for carrying out this activity: found in any sizable organization, the function is variously called a review, an audit, or an investigation.

From ancient times to the present, every individual in authority who must depend on others to do the work for which he is ultimately responsible is nagged by a suspicion that the information he is being given may not fully represent what is actually going on. This has led to the presence of review systems that operate independently of routine reporting and accounting procedures.

The process operates at several levels within the structure of government, and health agencies are no exception. The supervisor who regularly takes time to ride with the field staff is auditing the operation to see if the work being done corresponds to the information in the reports. The agency or division that maintains a review staff who report directly to the director is engaging in the same exercise.

Review, if well set up and carried out, contributes to program improvement. The results of a review done poorly range from a waste of time and resources to actual damage to the future of a program. Good or bad, however, reviews are a fact of life that can, often unexpectedly, directly involve any member of an organization. If employees have received no background orientation on the reasons for (and structure of) the review process, the normal reaction to being reviewed (a mixture of irritation, suspicion, and apprehension) may be heightened.

Reviews are conducted for several purposes and under a variety of terminologies. We will discuss the broad reviews concerned with program activity, which usually include some attention to economics as well as operations; we will not discuss routine financial audits.

175

Program reviews can be either periodic general examinations, which will be referred to as audits, or more narrowly focused studies resulting from a specific situation, which will be referred to as investigations. Program audits or investigations can be generated internally (within the operating agency) or externally (from a government level outside the operating agency).

## Internal Audits

A formal, general review group usually is created by an agency head to provide an independent look at program activities. Sometimes called an internal audit staff, or by a less forbidding title such as program appraisal or program review staff, the value of such a group to the organization depends on how the audit group is perceived and how its activities are structured and staffed.

A sound audit is nothing more than an unbiased comparison of what is being done to a prescribed standard. For an organization, the prescribed standard can only be the established policies, rules, and regulations under which the agency operates. A reviewer (auditor), or review staff that is allowed to substitute personal opinion for organizational policy produces a poor product, resentment in those under review, and invalid information for agency managers.

To be effective, a program review must be conducted in the field where the work is done. However, since the reviewers and those they interview are members of the same organization, it will be divisive if reviewers in the field are regarded as foreign interlopers. Discussing preliminary findings with the supervisor of the unit being audited is not only a courtesy but will also help detect errors that can be corrected before the final report is written.

Program audits are of no value unless they are studied and acted upon by the line management of the organization. Because an active program audit group generates a lot of paperwork, an administrative weakness is to delay acting on the reports. Slippage in this area, once it starts, tends to increase, and the audit process may come to be regarded as a nuisance. Results require a timely follow-up system to monitor implementation of corrective actions determined to be necessary.

Careful selection of program auditors is critical for an effective internal appraisal. Career professionals with broad experience in the organization should be sought. Since program audits provide an excellent means for learning how the total organization operates, above-average individuals who are dedicated to the work of the agency and who are expected to assume larger responsibilities in the future should be selected.

Auditors should also have the ability to meet and deal with people. The auditor will not get much information unless confidence and respect are quickly established to reduce or eliminate suspicion, which develops even under the best circumstances.

In comparison with most other work assignments, a program auditor is in an ideal situation. Direct access to the management structure gives an auditor considerable implied authority with no direct responsibility for producing program results. However, authority without responsibility is a potentially dangerous combination, and if assignment to a review staff becomes a comfortable permanent career, the danger is magnified. For this reason, as well as to provide the balance that comes from fresh viewpoints, review assignments should be for a limited time with carefully selected reviewers rotating through the appraisal staff and returning to the line responsibilities of the agency.

## Internal Investigations

A health agency is usually a unit of a larger department or ministry; thus, agency investigations may be limited to specific incidents confined to program operations. Instances concerned with violations of broader government regulations or rules or with suspected illegal practices are often relegated to the investigative arm of the department or ministry or to the judicial system. If a program involved in an investigation is being carried out in cooperation with another department, state, province, or country where the appropriate investigative responsibilities lie it may be affected by the terms of the agreement between the cooperating jurisdictions.

If the appropriate investigation of an incident lies within the authority of the program agency, many of the considerations discussed under internal audits are applicable. Each investigation is a special event, and the instructions and objectives for each investigation must be tailored to the situation. The investigator(s) selected must be sufficiently experienced in the activity concerned with the investigation to be able to make informed and objective recommendations.

In contrast to an ongoing internal program audit system, investigations are unpredictable and usually initiated in response to what may be a significant breach of prescribed procedure. No internal investigation should be carried out in secrecy. Anyone familiar with organizational culture knows that secrecy within an organization is an illusion, and attempts at secrecy only create adversarial attitudes between program management and the rest of the organization.

## External Audits

Externally generated audits, in contrast to those generated internally, reverse the focus of concern as far as the organization is concerned. Agency management justifiably feels that they are the ones under scrutiny, regardless of where within the agency the audit is being conducted. Field staff quickly recognize that any adverse comments by external auditors will reflect more on agency management than on themselves; thus, even an agency head who is a strong believer in the value of the internal review staff will look with some suspicion at audits imposed from outside, not stopping to think that the field staff may react similarly to the internal appraisals.

External and internal audits arise from the same base; concern by the legislative branch or higher levels within the executive branch that outside examination is useful in finding out what is really going on. Implementing this concern can take several forms. Within the federal structure of the United States, external review groups that occasionally conduct audits of animal health programs include special commissions appointed by the Department of Agriculture, legislative hearings conducted by congressional committees, in-depth studies by the Office of the President through the Office of Management and Budget (OMB), and program audits carried out by the General Accounting Office (GAO), an arm of Congress. Similar structures are found in many states within the United States as well as in other countries.

Within the federal structure the most frequent and comprehensive audits are carried out periodically by the GAO. In addition, the GAO may conduct special investigations as a result of specific requests from committees or members of Congress. Since most domestic animal health programs are carried out by the federal government in cooperation with the states, a GAO review involving these programs is also of considerable interest to the states. Industries directly affected by veterinary regulatory responsibilities pay close attention to GAO audits of the regulatory agencies. GAO auditors pride themselves in approaching their work objectively, even though an initial request for an audit may reflect a much narrower interest. It is obvious, however, that no audit is conducted with the aim of heaping praise on the target of the review. The purpose, unstated as it may be, is to search for deficiencies.

OMB examiners and their counterparts in state government or in other countries are concerned with protecting the top executive level of the government from inefficiency or unjustifiable fund requests by subordinate agencies. In recent years cost/benefit studies have become an important basis for the interchanges between such examiners and agencies under review. In contrast to GAO audits, executive branch reviews usually do not involve extensive field work, but largely depend on the examiners to challenge the data submitted by the agencies.

The nature of the whole process makes it inevitable that conflicting views arise between the auditors and the agency under review, and these conflicts usually center on differing definitions of reality. The external auditor usually comes from a different professional background, and regardless of how well that auditor tries to prepare for the study, the depth of understanding of the work will not be as great as the agency's, particularly for health related programs. It is the responsibility of the agency under review to provide full background information on its activities and to argue the agency's case strongly when differences arise. If this is not done and the final audit report contains unwarranted conclusions and recommendations, the fault lies as much with the agency as with the auditors.

## External Investigations

Special investigations of agency actions or personnel by outside investigators usually involve serious allegations of improper or illegal activities, ranging from misuse of vehicles or supplies, to misuse of funds, to bribery. These investigations are often initiated by the inspector general's office of the parent department or ministry and may expand to include the police and judicial systems. Special investigations usually involve individuals or small groups rather than an entire agency, although a comprehensive external investigation may result if the initial investigation discovers widespread improprieties within an agency. While the initial indication of improper activity often arises within the operating agency, investigation of this type is not usually a function of the program group.

## Maintaining Objectivity

Public organizations and public employees operate in the public eye and must realize that they will be under scrutiny whenever allegations are made against them, therefore, the environment to be sought is one that will promote an objective approach.

Definitions of objectivity, however, differ depending on the past experience and conditioning of the parties. Objectivity in internal reviews is subject to control by the agency management, whereas objectivity during external reviews is not under total control of the agency under review. However, the agency has an important responsibility in this area.

Many cooperative federal-state animal health programs operate under state authority within the state under joint memorandums of understanding. This makes it difficult for federal auditors without prior experience with shared authority to understand how the programs are conducted within a state. If the agency under review makes no effort to clarify the legal basis for the program, the auditors may come to inaccurate or unrealistic conclusions.

The complexities of diagnostic procedures or vaccines used in animal health programs, resulting from the variables inherent in dealing with biological systems, may be beyond the understanding of an auditor without a biological science background. Without scientific training, the auditor often may be looking for certainties, and may be unwilling to accept anything less than certainties, unless agency personnel clearly explain that those certainties cannot be expected when dealing with biological processes.

When international programs are involved, an auditor with only a national viewpoint may try to judge the work from only that frame of reference even though the program may be operating under a multinational agreement that spells out the basis of operation. One of the authors encountered this problem during the Mexican-U.S. campaign against foot-and-mouth disease in Mexico when U.S. auditors came to Mexico and tried to judge personnel and program activities by internal U.S. standards rather than by the terms of the agreement under which the joint Mexican-U.S. commission operated.

Public agencies, including those conducting health programs, will continue to be audited and/or investigated. Personnel who receive orientation in the audit and investigation systems learn what to expect if they become involved in a review. In addition, the broader the understanding by agency personnel of the historical, scientific, and regulatory foundations of their work, the more fully they will be able to answer inquiries during an audit or investigation.

# 24

# Analyzing Value

VALUE VARIES according to individual interests and biases; thus the value of a health program will not necessarily be viewed the same way by all parties at interest. In fact, a measured evaluation of the economic worth of a particular approach to disease control or eradication may differ from some perceived "self-evident" truths. The National Brucellosis Technical Commission (1978c) projected possible economic returns to consumers and producers from several alternative courses for conducting the brucellosis program. One of these involved adding to the existing basic program a system for high-level, whole-herd vaccination in areas of high prevalence. Over a 20-yr period it was projected that this could result in a return to consumers of $14 for every $1 invested. In contrast, producers would lose over $8 for every $1 they invested in program costs over the same period. This outcome, largely due to the potential for increased milk and beef supplies and resultant lower commodity prices, presumably would be dismaying to those producers who were insisting that an adult vaccination program was needed to keep them in business.

Most large-scale animal health programs are pursued because of economic loss from disease; economic analysis of the worth of the program or of comparative costs of carrying out the program is a valid management tool. In fact, current requirements in many political jurisdictions call for economic analyses as part of the planning and operational process. Health management professionals must develop an understanding of how this activity fits into the technical, political, and cultural factors that are also involved.

Economic analysis aims to evaluate the net economic worth of programs. A cattle producer can quickly decide whether or not to spend $500 to save a $300 cow, but a large regional or national program involves too many disparate economic factors to quickly reach a valid opinion on net return.

As economic return is the primary reason for engaging in the production of food and fiber animals, an optimal production plan often must be tempered to one that is merely adequate in order to show a profit. However, if economic analyses of alternative approaches find that a marginally adequate eradication program is the only alternative that can be shown as cost effective, serious questions should be asked as to the advisability of embarking on the campaign. Successful disease eradication cannot be assumed from a marginally adequate effort.

Another important value of good economic analyses is that they will be presented in terms that can be understood by individuals of varying backgrounds and thus serve as a common evaluating point for policymakers at all levels.

There are, of course, noneconomic reasons for pursuing animal health programs, particularly if actual or perceived threats to human health loom large in the public consciousness. Rabies is subject to prevention or control programs in animals because of the threat to human health. Anyone involved in the campaign to eradicate Venezuelan equine encephalomyelitis from the United States will remember that the general public reacted so strongly to the fear of human infection that it was possible to spray 13.5 million acres with insecticides for mosquito control with no significant opposition.

Generally, however, even in cases of animal disease where human health risk may also be present, the concern of livestock and poultry producers is primarily economic, and their support for animal health programs is due to economic factors. This is to be expected when dealing with domesticated species maintained for economic reasons.

## The Numbers Game

Numbers are a peculiarly human invention used to express succinctly even greater volumes of abstract thought, also a peculiarly human attribute. Most of us are aware of, and sometimes even use, mathematical expressions that we have learned but do not understand; e.g., Einstein's $E = mc^2$ is widely known but seldom grasped.

The proper use of numbers, then, lies not in memorizing the figures, or even the rules for their manipulation, but in evaluating the background represented by the numbers. This is even more important when machines do our calculations, machines that are not capable of abstract reasoning.

Sound analysis of the economic value of animal health programs does not depend on the volume of numbers expressed but on the validity of the facts and assumptions used to construct the numbers. Economists and statisticians, as with any fraternity of specialists, have their own catalogue of formulations that tends to confuse the uninformed and intimidate the uninitiated. The task of the health professional is to participate meaningfully in the analytical process to prevent the drawing of vast conclusions from inadequate information. Apropos to this point,

> It is an easy and fatal step to think that the accuracy of our arithmetic is equivalent to the accuracy of our knowledge about the problem in hand. We suffer from "delusions of accuracy." Once an enthusiast gets this dis-

ease, he and all who depend on his conclusions for their welfare are damned. (Monroney 1965)

No decisionmaker, including anyone responsible for health program management, should accept an economic analysis without a clear expression of the background material on which the conclusions are founded, or participate in developing such an analysis without insisting that any questionable numbers be thrown out. McCallon (1973) observed that if garbage is analyzed, the results will be garbage; guesswork, even if based on the only information available, is still guesswork and has no place in analysis.

This means that if acceptable information (numbers) on which to base an analysis is insufficient, the analysis should not be attempted unless and until supportable data are acquired.

We are currently in love with statistics. Advertisers try to find a way to introduce the word into their copy (statistics show that 9 out of 10, etc.) in order to create an illusion of authenticity or accuracy. Politicians are prone to use statistics to support the particular point they are espousing at the moment. None of these should be accepted as meaningful, of course, without a knowledge of how the numbers were constructed and, of equal importance, what may be omitted.

While statistical data are a necessary part of economic models, such data, as in any conclusion based on a degree of assumption, have varying levels of certainty, depending on how they are drawn. Monroney (1965) points out that statistical analysis, when properly conducted, is a delicate dissection of uncertainties, a surgery of suppositions. Informed respect, tempered with a measure of skepticism, is the attitude one should have toward the use of numerical data.

There are different types of statistics: descriptive statistics (those that summarize or describe data, such as the Agricultural Statistics published by the USDA) and inferential statistics (Beal 1975b). Inferential statistics are concerned with the analysis of data and the drawing of conclusions from this data and have considerable application in developing economic models for animal health programs.

While a competent statistician is needed to properly carry out the technical aspects of economic modeling for large-scale programs, it is important for the health professional to have a grasp of the basic concepts that must be followed to obtain information that can be used. For large populations, a sampling system is usually the only feasible way to gather valid information. In this context, it is well to again stress the basic necessity for sound sampling, which is randomization, i.e., drawing the sample so that each member of the population sampled has an equal chance of being included.

Truly random results may be difficult to obtain even when an entire population is presumably covered. In such cases some type of sensitivity check can be sought. Beal (1986) found correlation between falling hog cholera condemnation rates on federal antemortem and postmortem inspection and the widening ratio of confirmed cases to initially suspicious cases reported from the field. During the fiscal years 1964–1973, the bulk of U.S. swine were covered by both federal inspection at slaughter and by a compulsory hog cholera reporting system in the field; the comparative results reinforced the validity of the falling rate reported from the field program.

Reduction of the uncertainties always present in assembling data is one benefit from a cooperative effort between health professionals, biometricians, and economists, if each group understands the concepts under which the others operate.

## Benefit/Cost Analysis

A variety of groups, including those interested in disease control, are always competing for a portion of public funds: it is axiomatic that demands for public funds always exceed availability. In recent years, as a balance to the political avenues used in this competition, many national governments and international bodies have required benefit/cost analyses of proposed programs.

Obviously, no proposed program can expect support if the estimated costs far exceed the expected benefits. As estimates of benefits and effectiveness of a proposed program must be made in advance of the efforts, they must be based on some assumptions. These assumptions usually determine the outcome of the analysis and are critical to the study. Fortunately, the objectivity of these assumptions usually is maintained by review at many levels and by various agencies. In this review process, assumptions should be challenged and weaknesses exposed, so that the final result can be defended with reasonable objectivity from an economic standpoint and will provide a logical basis for obtaining support.

Beal (1975) points out that a benefit/cost analysis merely asks and answers the question of whether the cost of a particular activity is justified by the benefit to be obtained from that activity.

There are two basic techniques available to compare benefits and costs of alternative courses of action (National Brucellosis Technical Commission 1978c): the partial budgeting technique, in which the added benefits and cost to be accrued within a specified population are identified and estimated; and systems simulation, which attempts to model a simplified version of the "whole world" in order to better assess the impact of alternative actions on the total system. Systems simulation tries to go beyond a single element of a complicated total.

It is important for program management purposes to examine the effect of a program on a single industry or facet of an industry. However, it is also important for overall policy decisions between competing programs to gain some understanding of the benefits and costs of each for the broad spectrum of society.

Benefit/cost analyses, whether retrospective (analyzing what happened) or prospective (analyzing what may happen), always operate in the context of "compared to what?" Alternative routes of action are compared. Even in a retrospective analysis only one set of circumstances can actually have occurred. For example, Ellis (1972) used benefit/cost analytical techniques to evaluate the swine fever (hog cholera) eradication program completed several years previously in Great Britain. The actual effect of the eradication program was compared with what might have happened during the same years if the previously existing control program had been continued.

Prospective analyses are more in demand than retrospective analyses. Alternatives considered in such studies generally compare a no-change situation with one or more alternative programs. For example, McCauley et al. (1975), in the benefit/cost analysis portion of their study of the potential economic impact of foot-and-mouth disease (FMD) in the United States, considered three alternative responses should FMD be introduced into the United States. All were compared to a 15-yr base period (1976–1990) with the United States continuing free of FMD and preventive policies remaining in effect. The possible alternative responses, also measured over the same 15-yr period, were (1) endemic FMD with no public control programs, (2) endemic FMD with compulsory vaccination, and (3) eradication through a stamping-out program.

Sensitivity testing of benefit/cost ratios can be provided by changing some of the assumptions. Ellis (1972) considered two assumptions under the alternative of a continued swine fever control program in Great Britain. One, which he believed was the best supported, was for a further rise in incidence before any decline commenced, and the other projected a continuous decline in outbreaks. Eradication results, when compared with the first subalternative (control with initially rising incidence) showed a benefit/cost ratio of 4.03:1. When compared with the second (control with declining incidence) the ratio was 2.62:1; but in both cases eradication was the desirable program economically.

Benefit/cost analysis, as illustrated by these examples, involves (1) deciding on the alternative courses of action to be evaluated and compared, (2) constructing a model for each that aims to determine what might happen if the alternative was pursued through the time period selected, and (3) comparing the discounted benefits and costs that would result with each.

The concept is clear and orderly. The execution has increased in sophistication over recent years, as those in the field search for ways to improve the scope and validity of the background estimates on which the final results will be based. Assumptions are required, and as the outcome is largely dependent on these assumptions, the strength of an analysis comes from the soundness of those assumptions and the severity with which those assumptions are tested.

The final expression of benefit/cost analysis is that the benefits either do or do not exceed costs, but this figure does not give the background information on which the result is based. Anyone who needs the result as part of a decision or policy-making process should not accept the results without reviewing the entire presentation. In the early years of enthusiasm for this approach, assumptions were sometimes made that were improbable or poorly supported, producing results that were superficially attractive but unrealistic as a basis for decision making. McCallon (1973) points out that a perfectionist will never complete an economic model for he will continually be looking for more perfect information, and, as a good analyst, will prepare a model that can be readily changed when additional information becomes available.

One technical feature of economic modeling that will be new to many health professionals is the inclusion of what is referred to as discounting, which is necessary to properly compare the economic worth of the alternatives considered. The analysis of a health program must be projected over a number of years to be realistic, during which the value of money will change. Both sides of the equation (benefits and costs) must be discounted back to the present value; in other words, building in the "interest" income that would have been available if the savings (benefits) and expenses (costs) had been used for other purposes. This is of significance for decisionmakers at levels that require comparisons of the worth of the various projects competing for funds.

It is obvious that the annual discount rate used in the calculations can affect the final comparative worth of the alternatives considered; therefore, the discount rate selected should be realistic. Sensitivity testing for this factor frequently includes comparing several discount rates.

Large publicly funded animal health programs consume resources that otherwise would be available for other public purposes, and it is obvious that the economic worth of a proposed program will be judged on not only whether it returns more than it costs, but also how that rate of return compares with use of the same funds for other purposes. Various agencies seeking support for their projects will be preparing benefit/cost studies; the decisionmakers look to these studies as an economic common denominator on which to make judgments.

Those involved in the process should remember that final decisions on public programs are made on the basis of many factors, only one of which is economic worth. Economic analysis is a valuable tool in the process at both the program agency level and at higher policy levels. For the program agency the value of the process goes beyond economics, as a sound analysis requires examination of all the factors that go into the conduct of a program.

## Cost Effectiveness and Operational Options

Regardless of the political, cultural, and economic factors involved in deciding to initiate an animal health program, the operating agency will be expected to produce the desired results efficiently. Efficiency will be equated with cost.

Comparing the cost of alternative methods that can be used to produce the same benefits is the study of cost effectiveness (Plumb 1983). The analysis is thus operationally oriented and focuses more narrowly than benefit/cost analyses.

When the United States decided it would be desirable to send a manned flight to the moon, the goal was fixed. A cost analysis of the various flight systems that would achieve the goal would have been a cost-effectiveness study. If it had been decided to do a broad economic analysis of whether such an achievement would be economically beneficial to the society, that study, combined with the cost-effectiveness results of the operational alternatives, would have been a benefit/cost analysis.

Although cost-effectiveness studies are a necessary part of the benefit/cost analysis for any public program, such studies are also important as part of the operational management of a program. This includes studying the cost effectiveness of significant program changes that may be contemplated, as well as for new programs still in the planning stage.

Cost-effectiveness studies, being relatively narrow in focus, can deal with fewer uncertainties and assumptions than a simulation model of a larger universe. However, analysis for cost effectiveness, even though it may deal with fewer abstractions and uncertainties than a benefit/cost study, is a time consuming process when properly performed. McCallon (1973) states that the various inputs of the program being considered need to be divided into the smallest units practicable (so that over-estimates in one may be balanced by under-estimates in another) and that a flow chart of all program activities (through which the program can be run on a step-by-step basis) is useful.

Analyzing value in a structured fashion, for any program, is heavily dependent on the principle that an aggregate answer based on detailed examination of individual uncertainties will be better than a single all-encompassing conclusion based on a few large assumptions.

It is beyond the scope of this volume to attempt a manual on the techniques of economic analysis. A number of economic analyses of animal health programs have been published, including several references cited in this chapter.

# REFERENCES

Adlam, G. H. 1979. Planning and implementation of disease control programs—experience in New Zealand. Proc. 2d. Int. Symp. Vet. Epidemiol. Econ. Canberra, Austr. May.

American Veterinary Medical Association. 1978 and 1986. Reports of the AVMA panel on euthanasia. 173:59–72 and 188:252–68.

———. 1983. Veterinary Economic Statistics. Office of Economics. Schaumberg, Ill.: AVMA.

Anderson, R. M.; Jackson, H. C.; May, R. M.; and Smith, A. M. 1981. Population dynamics of fox rabies in Europe. Nature 289:765–71.

Arnstein, P.; Eddie, B.; and Meyer, K. F. 1968. Control of psittacosis by group chemotherapy of infected parrots. Am. J. Vet. Res. 29:2213–27.

Audy, J. R. 1958. The localization of disease with special reference to the zoonoses. Trans. Roy. Soc. Trop. Med. Hyg. 52:305–34.

Aulaqi, N. A. 1979. Cost evaluation of alternative carcass disposal methods in disease eradication programs. Potential Economic Impact of Foot-and-Mouth Disease in the United States. Tech. Rep. No. 4. Univ. of Minnesota.

Aulaqi, N. A., and Sundquist, W. B. 1979. Indemnification under animal disease control programs with special emphasis on foot-and-mouth disease. Potential Economic Impact of Foot-and-Mouth Disease in the United States. Tech. Rep. No. 12. Univ. of Minnesota.

Axnick, N. W., and Lane, J. M. 1972. Costs associated with the protection of the United States against smallpox. World Health Organization offset document, WHO/SE/72, 45. Geneva.

Baltazard, M. 1960. Déclin et destin d'une maladie infectieuse: La peste. Bull. World Health Org. 23:247–62.

Barnett, L. 1948. The Universe and Dr. Einstein. New York: Harper and Row.

Bartlett, D. E. 1978. Marketing cattle semen on the continent. XI Inter-Am. Meet. Foot-and-Mouth Dis. Zoonoses Control. Pan Am. Health Org. Washington, D.C.

Bartlett, M. S. 1960. The critical community size for measles in the United States. J. Roy. Stat. Soc. Ser. A 123:37–44.

Beal, V. C.; Jr. 1975a. Considerations of sampling in regulatory veterinary medicine. In Regulatory Statistics. 5th. ed., Part III, Tables 1, 3. Washington, D.C.: Vet. Services, APHIS, USDA.

———. 1975b. Statistics—their use in animal disease eradication and control. In Regulatory Statistics. 5th. ed., Part I. Washington, D.C.: Vet. Services, APHIS, USDA.

———. 1986. Problems in interpreting animal disease data. Fallacies from biased data and biased interpretations. In Regulatory Statistics. 2d. ed., Vol. 2A, Part X. Washington, D.C.: Vet Services, APHIS, USDA.

Beran, G. W., and Gregorio, S. B. 1966. Sociological problems in a rabies control program in a community in the Philippines. Natl. Rabies Symp. Natl. Commun. Dis. Cent. Atlanta, Ga. May.

Bers, J. F. 1973. Airborne Transmission and Airborne Infections: Concepts and Methods. Proc. Int. Symp. Aerobiol. New York: Halstead.

Biberstein, E. L.; Cameron, H. S.; and Meyer, M. E. 1961. Brucella whey reaction in problem herds. J. Am. Vet. Assoc. 138:244–47.

Bierer, B. W. [1939] 1974. History of Animal Plagues of North America. Reprint. Washington, D.C.: USDA.

Brilliant, L. B., and Hodakevic, L. N. 1978. Certification of smallpox eradication. Bull. World Health Org. 56:723–33.

Burridge, M. J., and Schwabe, C. W. 1977. Epidemiological analysis of factors influencing rate of progress in *Echinococcus granulosus* control in New Zealand. J. Hyg. (Cambridge) 78:151–63.

Callis, J. J., and Shahan, M. S. 1970. Foot-and-mouth disease. In Diseases of Swine, 3rd ed. Ed. H. W. Dunne. Ames: Iowa State Univ. Press.

Canada Dept. of Agriculture. 1881–1905. Annual Reports of Chief Inspector of Stock.

_____. 1967. Canada Agriculture, the First 100 Years.

Carrizo, A., and Nelson, W. Q. 1976. Letter from COPFA to Federal Highway Commission. Panama City, Panama. March.

Center for Disease Control. 1979a. Texas man survives last U.S. smallpox. Dateline, Atlanta, Ga. 11:2.

_____. 1979b. U.S. saved dollars by "pox" demise. Dateline, Atlanta, Ga. 11:15.

_____. 1979c. Global effort pays off. Smallpox at target "zero." Dateline, Atlanta, Ga. 11:1–11.

Chaffee, S. H. 1972. The interpersonal context of mass communication. In Current Perspectives in Mass Communications Research. Ed. F. G. Kline and P. J. Tichenor. Beverly Hills, Calif.: Sage.

Chain, P. 1979. Public participation and communications in Latin American disease control programs. Proc. 2d. Int. Symp. Vet. Epidemiol. Econ. Canberra, Austr. May.

Chestnut, H. 1965. Systems Engineering Tools. New York: John Wiley.

Christiansen, K. H. 1979. Laboratory management and disease surveillance informaiton systems. Proc. 2d. Int. Symp. Vet. Epidemiol. Econ. Canberra, Austr. May.

Christiansen, K. H., and Hellstorm, J. S. 1979. The collection of data from New Zealand abattoirs and slaughter houses. Proc. 2d. Int. Symp. Vet. Epidemiol. Econ. Canberra, Austr. May.

Cockrill, W. R. 1963. The changing status of animal quarantine. Brit. Vet. J. 119:338–99.

Cohen, A. R. 1964. Act, Attitude Change and Social Influence. New York: Basic Books.

Dept. of Primary Industry. 1979. Bovine tuberculosis and brucellosis eradication in Australia 1977–78. Austr. Bur. Anim. Health. Canberra.

Diamant, G. 1978. Regulatory veterinary medicine. J. Am. Vet. Med. Assoc. 172:1.

Doby, P. B.; Schnurrenberger, P. R.; Martin, R. J.; Hanson, L. E.; Sherrick, G. W.; and Schoenholz, W. K. 1966. Western encephalitis in Illinois horses and ponies. J. Am. Vet. Med. Assoc. 148:402–26.

Doyle, K. A. 1979. The economic relevance of disease status and its definition, the national value of quarantine measures to protect livestock resources. Proc. 2d. Int. Symp. Vet. Epidemiol. Econ. Canberra, Austr. May.

Ellis, P. R. 1972. An economic evaluation of the swine fever eradication programme in Great Britain. Dept. of Agric., Study 311. Univ. of Reading.

Elrick and Lovidge, Inc. 1961. Opportunities to increase the incidence of hog cholera immunization. Market research study for the Hog Cholera Control Agency.

Fekadu, M.; Shaddock, J. H.; and Baer, G. M. 1981. Intermittent excretion of rabies virus in the saliva of a dog two and six months after it had recovered from experimental rabies. Am. J. Trop. Med. Hyg. 30:1113–15.

Flagle, C. D. 1963. Operational research in the health services. Ann. N.Y. Acad. Sci. 107:748-59.

Foege, W. H.; Miller, J. D.; and Henderson, D. A. 1975. Smallpox eradication in West and Central Africa. Bull. World Health Org. 52:209-22.

Foege, W. H.; Miller, J. D.; and Lane, J. M. 1971. Selective epidemiologic control in smallpox eradication. Am. J. Epidemiol. 94:311-15.

Gelfand, H. M. 1973. Concepts of disease eradication and control. 15th. Annu. Midwest Interprof. Semin. Dis. Common Anim. Man. Urbana, Ill. August.

Gordon, J. E. 1963. Changing accents in community disease. Am. J. Public Health 53:141-47.

Gorham, W. 1967. PBBS, its scope and limits. Public Interest 8:4.

Hagan, W. A. 1958. The control and eradication of animal diseases in the United States. Annu. Rev. Microbiol. 12:127-44.

Hanlon, J. H., and Pickett, G. E. 1979. Public Health: The Administration and Practice. St. Louis, Mo.: C. V. Cosby.

Henricson, D. A. 1976. The eradication of smallpox. Sci. Am. 235:25-33.

Henricson, W. 1975. Problems of government production and utilization of information on animal diseases. In Animal Disease Monitoring. Ed. D. E. Ingram, W. R. Mitchell, and S. W. Martin. Springfield, Ill.: Charles C. Thomas.

Hinman, E. H. 1966. World Eradication of Infectious Diseases. Springfield, Ill.: Charles C. Thomas.

Holden, C. 1978. Outbreak of equine VD stirs fear in Kentucky. Science 200:181-84.

Hubbert, W. T.; McCulloch, W. F.; and Schnurrenberger, P. R., eds. 1975. Diseases Transmitted from Animals to Man. Springfield, Ill.: Charles C. Thomas.

Hudson, R. S. 1983. Maintaining health, not preventing disease. In Principles of Health Maintenance. Ed. P. R. Schnurrenberger and R. S. Sharman. Philadelphia: Praeger.

Hugh-Jones, M. E.; Ellis, P. R.; and Felton, M. R. 1976. The use of a computer model of brucellosis in the dairy herd. In New Techniques in Veterinary Epidemiology and Economics. Ed. P. R. Ellis, A. P. M. Shaw, and A. J. Stephens. Reading, Eng.: Univ. of Reading Press.

Hutton, N. E. 1975. Computerized disease accounting systems for diagnostic laboratories. In Animal Disease Monitoring. Ed. D. E. Ingram, W. R. Mitchell, and S. W. Martin. Springfield, Ill.: Charles C. Thomas.

Johnson, B. G. 1982. Status of cooperative state-federal brucellosis eradication program. 83rd. Annu. Proc. U.S. Anim. Health Assoc.

Konyha, L. D. 1978. Epidemiologic principles in the bovine tuberculosis eradication program. Proc. Vet. Prev. Med. Epidemiol. Work Conf. Ames, Iowa. June.

Leakey, R. E., and Lewin, R. 1977. Origins: What New Discoveries Reveal About the Emergence of Our Species and Its Possible Future. New York: Dutton.

Leech, F. B. 1979. Relations between objectives and observations in epidemiological studies. Proc. 2d. Int. Symp. Vet. Epidemiol. Econ. Canberra. Austr. May.

McCallon, B. R. 1973. Determining the economic feasibility of a disease control program. In Animal Disease Eradication: Evaluating Programs. Madison: Univ. of Wisconsin.

McCauley, E. H.; Aulaqi, N. A.; New, J. C.; Sundquist, W. B.; and Miller, W. M. 1979. A Study of the Potential Impact of Foot-and-Mouth Disease in the United States. Tech. Bull. No. 1597. Univ. of Minnesota.

McClanaghan, R. J. 1961. Canada's hog cholera eradication program. In Symposium on Hog Cholera, Univ. of Minnesota.

McKeller, W. M. 1942. Cattle tick fever. In Keeping Livestock Healthy. Yearbook of Agriculture. Washington, D.C.: Government Printing Office.

Manthei, C. A.; Kuttler, A. K.; and Goode, E. R. 1956. Brucellosis. In Animal Diseases. Yearbook of Agriculture. Washington, D.C.: Government Printing Office.

Merchant, I. A. 1940. Veterinary Bacteriology. Ames: Iowa State College Press.

Miller, A. W. 1942. Sheep scab and its control. In Keeping Livestock Healthy. Yearbook of Agriculture. Washington, D.C.: Government Printing Office.

Miller, R. J. 1973. Cultural practices and disease control programs. In Animal Disease Eradication: Evaluating Programs. Madison: Univ. of Wisconsin.

Miller, W. M. 1976. A state-transition model of epidemic foot-and-mouth disease. In New Techniques in Veterinary Epidemiology and Economics. Ed. P. R. Ellis, A. P. M. Shaw, and A. J. Stephens. Reading, Eng.: Univ. of Reading Press.

Mohler, J. R. 1924. Foot-and-mouth disease, with special reference to the outbreak of 1914. U.S. Dept. of Agriculture Circular 325.

Monroney, M. J. [1951] 1965. Facts from Figures. Reprint. Great Britain: Penguin Books.

Montgomery, R. E. 1921. On a form of swine fever occurring in British East Africa (Kenya Colony). J. Comp. Pathol. Ther. 34:159–91, 243–62.

Moore, C. G., and Schnurrenberger, P. R. 1981. A review of naturally occurring *Brucella abortus* infections in wild mammals. J. Am. Vet. Med. Assoc. 179:1105–12.

Morris, R. S., and Roe, R. T. 1975. The use of computer simulation in the design, evaluation, and monitoring of animal disease control programs. In Animal Disease Monitoring. Ed. D. G. Ingram, W. R. Mitchell, and S. W. Martin. Springfield, Ill.: Charles C. Thomas.

Mussman, H. C.; McCallun, W.; and Otte, E. 1979. Planning and implementation of animal disease control programs in developing countries. Proc. 2d. Int. Symp. Vet. Epidemiol. Econ. Canberra, Austr. May.

National Brucellosis Technical Commission. 1978a. Report. Washington, D.C.: APHIS, USDA. August.

———. 1978b. The Public Health Aspects of Brucellosis. Appendix A, Table 3, A-43. Washington, D.C.: APHIS, USDA. August.

———. 1978c. Benefit-Cost Analysis. Appendix B, B-163. Washington, D.C.: APHIS, USDA. August.

National Cancer Institute. 1969. Standard Veterinary Nomenclature for Diseases and Operations. Bethesda, Maryland.

Naylor, T. H.; Balintfly, G. L.; Burdick, D. S.; and Chu, K. 1966. Computer Simulation Techniques. New York: John Wiley and Sons.

Pavlovsky, E. N. 1966. Natural Nidality of Transmissible Diseases, with Special Reference to the Landscape Epidemiology of Zooanthroposes (in Russian). Urbana, Ill.: Univ. of Illinois Press.

Pinkus, C. E. 1968. A proposal for federal regulations of primate importation and disease contol. Int. Symp. Health Aspects Int. Movement Anim. Pan Am. Health Org. 182. Washington, D.C.

Plommet, M.; Renoux, G.; Philippon, A.; Gestin, J.; and Fensterbank, R. 1971. Transmission concentrate de la brucelose bovine d'une generation a l'autre. Bull. Acad. Vet. 44:53–59.

Plumb, J. A. 1983. Principles of Health Maintenance. Ed. P. R. Schnurrenberger and R. S. Sharman. New York: Praeger.

Ray, W. C. 1980. Recordkeeping and computer applications. Proc. Vet. Med. Epidemiol. Work Conf. Ft. Worth, Tex. February.

Roe, R. T. 1979. Features of the Australian national animal disease information system. Proc. 2d. Int. Symp. Vet. Epidemiol. Econ. Canberra, Austr. May.

Ross, J. E. 1973. Information, government programs and the public. In Animal Disease Eradication: Evaluating Programs. Madison: Univ. of Wisconsin.

Schnurrenberger, L. W. 1978. Epidemiological aspects of pseudorabies. Proc. Vet. Prev. Med. Epidemiol. Work Conf. Ames, Iowa. June.

Schnurrenberger, P. R., and Hubbert, W. T. 1981. Correlation between laboratory services and reporting requirements for selected zoonoses. Public Health Rep. 96:162–65.

Schnurrenberger, P. R.; Martin, R. J.; and Doby, P. B. 1965. Disease control through the study of population characteristics. Proc. U.S. Livest. Assoc. 69:29–34.

Schwabe, C. W. 1969. Veterinary Medicine and Human Health. Baltimore: Williams and Wilkins.

Sharman, E. C. 1978. Increasing complexities of importing and exporting livestock. Proc. Vet. Prev. Med. Epidemiol. Work Conf. Ames, Iowa. June.

Smith, A. W. 1984. Vesicular exanthema of swine and related caliciviral diseases. In Foreign Animal Diseases. Richmond, Va.: Contract printing for USAHA.

Smithcors, C. F. 1957. Evolution of the Veterinary Art. Kansas City, Mo.: Veterinary Medicine Publishing Co.

_____. 1963. The American Veterinary Profession. Ames: Iowa State Univ. Press.

Snyder, R. 1942. Cattle scab and its control. In Keeping Livestock Healthy. Yearbook of Agriculture. Washington, D.C.: Government Printing Office.

Soper, F. L. 1963. The elimination of urban yellow fever in the Americas through the eradication of Aedes aegypti. Am. J. Public Health. 53:7–16.

Steele, J. H. 1975. The development of disease surveillance: Its uses in disease control that relate to public and animal health. In Animal Disease Monitoring. Ed. D. E. Ingram, W. R. Mitchell, and S. W. Martin. Springfield, Ill.: Charles C. Thomas.

Stringfellow, D. A.; Howell, V. L.; and Schnurrenberger, P. R. 1982. Investigations into the potential for embryo transfer from Brucella abortus infected cows without transmission of infection. Theriogenology 18:733–43.

Todd, F. A. 1949. Developments in the regulatory control of animal disease in Germany. J. Am. Vet. Med. Assoc. 115:81–86.

_____. 1958. Defense against imported animal diseases. Adv. Vet. Sci. 4:1–50.

Traum, J. 1934. Foot-and-mouth disease, specific treatment, eradication, and differential diagnosis. Proc. 12th. Int. Vet. Congr. 2:87.

U.S. Animal Health Association. 1972–1984. Reports of the Committee on Livestock Identification. Annu. Proc.

_____. 1982. Report of the Committee on Parasitic Disease and Parasiticides. 86th. Annu. Proc.

U.S. Department of Agriculture. 1880. Report of the Commissioner of Agriculture.

_____. 1892. Report to the President.

_____. 1962. History of Hog Cholera Research in the U.S. Department of Agriculture 1884–1960. Agric. Inf. Bull. 1:241.

_____. 1973. Animal Protein Conservation. Work Group Report. Vet. Services, APHIS. Washington, D.C.

_____. 1978. Eradication of Exotic Newcastle Disease in Southern California 1971–1974. APHIS. Washington, D.C.

_____. 1981. Hog Cholera and Its Eradication. APHIS. Washington, D.C.

U.S. Livestock Sanitary Association. 1964. Foreign Animal Diseases.

Watt, G. E. L. 1979. Studies in the development of an abattoir traceback system for sheep. Proc. 2d. Int. Symp. Vet. Epidemiol. Econ. Canberra, Austr. May.

Wells, K. F. 1968. Disease problems associated with the importation and exportation of food animals and animal products. 3. The Canadian Viewpoint. Int. Symp. Health Aspects Int. Movement Anim. Pan Am. Health Org. 182. Washington, D.C.

_____. 1978. Technical aspects to consider in legislating for trade in products of animal origin between countries free of and infected by foot-and-mouth disease. XI Inter-Am. Meet. Foot-and-Mouth Dis. Zoonoses Control. Pan Am. Health Org. Washington, D.C.

Wilesmith, J. W., and Lorenz, R. J. 1979. Observations of the effects of farm husbandry and management factors on the prevalence and control of bovine leukosis virus infection in West Germany. Proc. 2d. Int. Symp. Vet. Epidemiol. Econ. Canberra, Austr. May.

Willeberg, P. E. 1979. Epidemiological applications of Danish swine slaughter inspection data. Proc. 2d. Int. Symp. Vet. Epidemiol. Econ. Canberra, Austr. May.

Yorke, J. A.; Nathanson, N.; Pianigiani, G.; and Martin, J. 1979. Seasonality and the requirements for perpetuation of viruses in populations. Am. J. Epidemiol. 190:103–22.

# INDEX